Imaging of the Cervical Spine in Children

Leonard E. Swischuk

Imaging of the Cervical Spine in Children

Second Edition

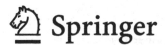

Leonard E. Swischuk, MD
Department of Pediatric Radiology
University of Texas Medical Branch
Galveston, TX, USA

ISBN 978-1-4939-4146-9   ISBN 978-1-4614-3788-8 (e-book)
DOI 10.1007/978-1-4614-3788-8
Springer New York Heidelberg Dordrecht London

Printed on acid-free paper

Springer is part of Springer Science+Business Media (www.springer.com)

To Janie, my wife
my life, my love, and my anchor
for over fifty years

Preface

When I first got into Pediatric Radiology in the 1960s and then when I moved to UTMB in Galveston, Texas in 1970, I became more and more interested in the cervical spine. I realized that in the pediatric age group, interpretation of the cervical spine images was often a problem for everyone, including myself. The reason for this was that there are many normal physiologic and anatomic variations that frequently mimic pathology, and at times this would become confusing.

Fortunately, shortly after arriving in Galveston, I came across a monograph entitled *The Upper Cervical Spine,* authored in 1972 by Detlef von Torklus and Walter Gehle from the orthopedic clinic and outpatient department at University Hospital in Hamburg Germany. This book was excellent in explaining anatomic and physiologic phenomena and was of great help for me. I then went on to look at things such as physiologic subluxation of C2 on C3, wedging of C3 and C4, the predental distance, and the differences in fractures sustained under the age of 5 from those sustained in older children and adults. Slowly, I began to feel more comfortable with the C-Spine and started to publish articles on it and also write chapters and textbooks. To this date, the lectures that I am asked to do most often are "The Cervical Spine: What Is Normal and What Is Abnormal," and another lecture on the same topic with a slightly different title, "The Cervical Spine in Children: When to Worry?"

Although all of this started with plain films, many of the findings are now readily transferable to CT and MR, especially Sagittal reconstructed views on CT. Therefore, I have attempted to blend the findings on plain films with those seen on CT and MR and emphasize which imaging modality produces best results, for any given condition. In addition, there is constant emphasis on normal anatomic and physiologic phenomena that mimic pathology.

Finally, I would like to thank my secretary Shirl Veal for all her assistance with this book. She is always up to any challenge and performs her duties with expertise and promptness. I am indebted to her for all the help she has given me in preparing this book.

Galveston, TX, USA   Leonard E. Swischuk, MD

Contents

Developmental Anatomy

The third through seventh vertebrae of the cervical spine are similar in their development, but development is different for the first and second vertebrae. All the cervical vertebrae develop from primitive sclerotomes [1], but the upper cervical spine, because of its functional complexity evolves from both the occipital and upper cervical sclerotomes (Fig. 1.1). These sclerotomes undergo significant embryologic alterations so as to eventually be able to accommodate free movement of the head on the first two (atlas and axis) cervical vertebrae. In this regard, the skull first must sit firmly on the atlas. This is accomplished by way of the occipital condyles articulating with the lateral masses of C1. This union is ensured by the presence of strong ligaments between these two structures. Thereafter, the skull and C1 must be able to rotate freely on C2. This is facilitated by the dens, which serves as a pivot for this function. The resultant rotatory movement occurs primarily at the C1–C2 level, but it should be underscored that while C1 rotates, within limits, around the dens, on *flexion and extension, the skull, C1, and C2 move as a unit.*

In terms of the derivation of the various portions of the upper cervical spine from the primitive sclerotomes, the atlas (C1) is derived from the first cervical sclerotome (Fig. 1.1). The axis (C2) is derived from the second cervical sclerotome. This sclerotome gives rise to the body, lateral masses, and neural arch of C2, *but not the dens. The dens actually is the body of C1* and as such is derived from the first cervical sclerotome. *The ossicle at the tip of the dens (the os terminale)* *is derived from the fourth occipital sclerotome (specifically known as the proatlas).* The dens itself arises from two primordial centers, which eventually fuse with the os terminale to form the mature dens (Fig. 1.2). If they remain separate the dens often is referred to as bifid, but still normal (see Fig. 4.19)

In terms of the development of the third through seventh cervical vertebra, and actually the body and neural arch of C2, there are six chondrofication centers [2]. These are diagrammatically depicted in Fig. 1.3, and while in most cases all these centers unite, if they fail to unite or develop, predictable anomalous configurations result. For example, if the two vertebral body centers fail to completely unite, a sagittal cleft vertebra results (Fig. 1.3b). If the union of the two vertebral body chondrofication centers is more advanced, but yet incomplete, a so-called butterfly vertebra develops (see Fig. 3.1), and when one or other, or both, of the vertebral body chondrofication centers fail to develop, a hemivertebra, or absence of a vertebra, results (Fig. 1.3c, d). Failure of development of the midchondrofication center leads to the absence of the pedicle (Fig. 1.3e), and if failure of the chondrofication center of the neural arch occurs, partial or complete absence of the neural arch results (Fig. 1.3f, g). Finally, if the two neural arches fail to unite posteriorly, a spina bifida results (Fig. 1.3h). However, development of the vertebral bodies at this stage is not complete for later, two vertebral body ossification centers develop. One is ventral and the other dorsal

L.E. Swischuk, *Imaging of the Cervical Spine in Children*,
DOI 10.1007/978-1-4614-3788-8_1, © Springer Science+Business Media New York 2013

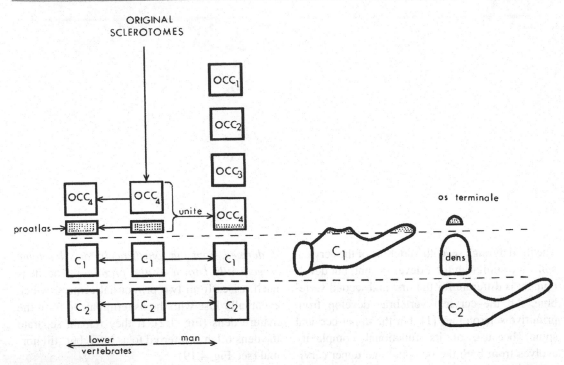

Fig. 1.1 Embryologic development of the upper cervical spine. The skull and upper cervical spine develop from primitive sclerotomes; the skull from occipital sclerotomes and the spine from upper cervical sclertomes. The occipital sclerotomes tend to fuse and reduce in number which often is accompanied by deletion of some of their more primordial elements. It is important to note, however, that the primitive proatlas prevails and unites with the primordial fourth occipital sclerotome to form the final occipital sclerotome. The os terminale is derived from this sclerotome. The first vertebral body (C1) is derived from the first cervical sclerotome. The dens actually is the body of C1, but eventually it unites with the body of C2, which is derived from the second cervical sclerotome

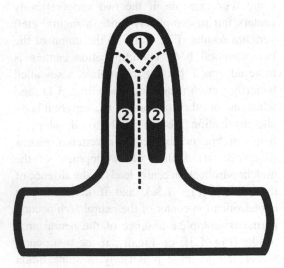

Fig. 1.2 Ossification centers of the dens. Note the two centers (2) for the body of the dens and the single center (1) for the tip, or os terminale

(Fig. 1.4a). If the ossification centers develop but fail to fuse, a coronal cleft vertebra results (Fig. 1.4b). If one or other of these ossification centers fails to develop, a coronal hemivertebra results (Fig. 1.4c, d). If both ossification centers fail to develop, the vertebral body will be hypoplastic or absent. Failure of the ossification centers of the neural arches to develop results in anomalies similar to those seen when the corresponding chondrofication centers fail to develop.

Normal Synchondroses

In the atlas (C1), normal synchondroses occur posteriorly through the spinous tip and anteriorly on either side of the central ossification center of

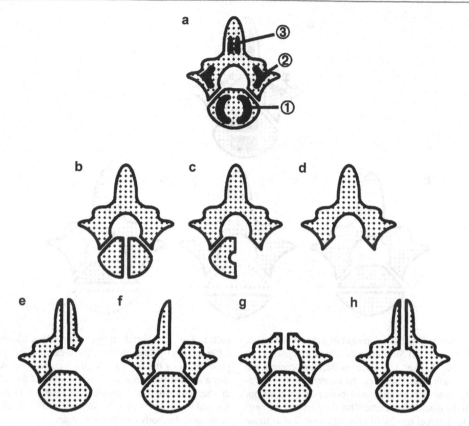

Fig. 1.3 Embryologic development of the cervical spine, chondrofication stage. (**a**) Note three chondrofication centers on each side: body (1), pars (2), and neural arch (3). (**b**) Lack of union of the body centers results in a sagittal cleft (complete), or butterfly (incomplete) vertebra. (**c**) Sagittal hemivertebra resulting from failure of development of one of the vertebral body centers. (**d**) Absent the anterior arch (Fig. 1.5). However, the anterior vertebra. Failure of development of both body centers. (**e**) Defect of pars. The center for the pars interarticularis fails to develop. (**f**) Lack of one center for the posterior arch usually results in half of the neural arch being present. (**g**) Absence of both posterior arch centers resulting in absence of the posterior arch. (**h**) Incomplete union of posterior arch (spina bifida)

the anterior arch (Fig. 1.5). However, the anterior arch of C1 is prone to multiple other synchondrotic defects [3] and as a result can assume a wide variety of configurations (Fig. 1.6). None of these should be misinterpreted as representing a "Jefferson fracture." Synchondroses generally have smooth edges with sclerotic margins. Occasionally the edges maybe a little irregular, but they still are smooth. True fractures show thin, sharp bony edges which lack smooth, sclerotic margins.

In the axis (C2), a synchondrosis is present between the dens and the body, and additionally on either side, between the body and dens and the body and neural arches (Figs. 1.7 and 1.8). On plain films the synchondrosis between the dens and the body is best visualized on lateral views of the cervical spine (Fig. 1.9a) and of course is vividly demonstrated with computerized tomography (Fig. 1.9c). This synchondrosis slowly closes as the individual enters childhood (Fig. 1.9d), but in infancy it can be quite wide (Fig. 1.9b). Anomalous and remnant synchondroses also can occur and often are best visualized with computerized tomography. They should not be misinterpreted as fractures (Fig. 1.10).

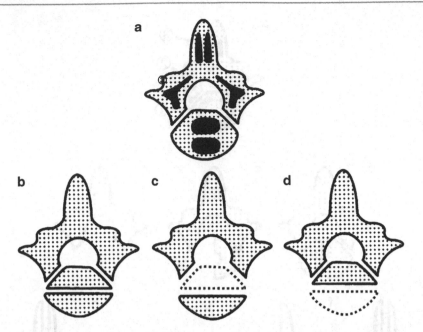

Fig. 1.4 Embryologic development of the cervical spine, ossification stage. (**a**) Similar to the chondrofication centers illustrated in Fig. 1.3, three ossification centers are present on each side. However, the centers for the vertebral body now are anterior and posterior in position. Failure of the ossification centers for the pars and the neural arch to develop results in anomalies similar to those seen in Fig. 1.3. Vertebral body anomalies, however, are different. (**b**) Coronal cleft vertebra resulting from incomplete union of the body ossification centers. (**c**) Anterior coronal hemivertebra results from failure of development of the posterior body ossification center. (**d**) Posterior coronal hemivertebra results from failure of development of the anterior body ossification center

The synchondroses between the neural arch and body of C2 are anterior in location, and on plain films are seen only on oblique views [4]. These synchondroses should not be misinterpreted as fractures, and in this regard, it is the synchondrosis between the dens and the neural arch of C2 that most likely suggests a fracture (Fig. 1.11a). A similar problem arises on far, parasagittal reconstructed computerized tomography slices (Fig. 1.11b, c).

In the third through seventh vertebrae, synchondroses occur anteriorly between the neural arches and the vertebral bodies (Fig. 1.12a).

On plain films they appear as defects between the lateral aspects of the vertebral bodies and the adjacent neural arches (Fig. 1.12b). Later, as they near fusion, they can appear as pseudofractures on oblique views of the cervical spine, but there should be no problem with correct diagnosis for they will be present in every vertebra (Fig. 1.12c).

Spina bifida (usually occulta), resulting from lack of posterior fusion of the neural arch, is more common in the lower cervical spine (Fig. 1.13a). Even though the resulting defect may be large (Fig. 1.13b, c), it is usually clinically nonconsequential.

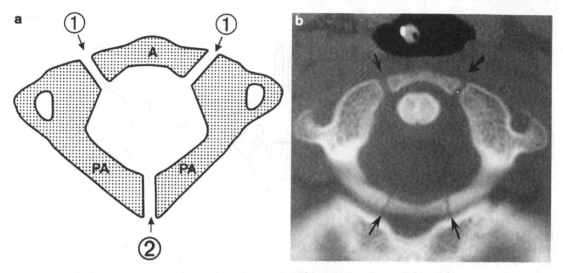

Fig. 1.5 Synchondroses of C1. (**a**) Diagrammatic representation of the usual anterior arch synchondroses (1) and normal posterior arch synchondrosis (2); anterior arch (A), posterior arch (PA). (**b**) Axial CT study showing the same anterior synchondroses (*anterior arrows*). In this patient there also are two anomalous, posterior synchondroses (*posterior arrows*)

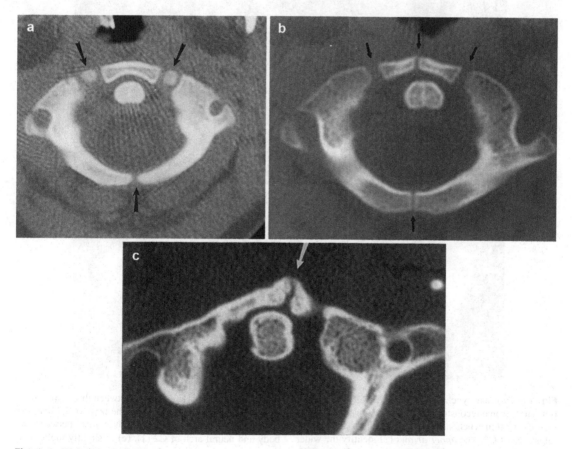

Fig. 1.6 Variable synchondrotic configurations of C1. (**a**) Two extra ossicles (*anterior arrows*) are present in this patient. Also note the posterior synchondrosis through the posterior neural arch (*posterior arrow*). (**b**) Three separate anterior synchondroses are present (*arrows*) in this individual. Normal posterior arch synchondrosis (*posterior arrow*). (**c**) This synchondrosis (*arrow*) in an adult is accompanied by dysplastic and hypertrophic degenerative bone formation

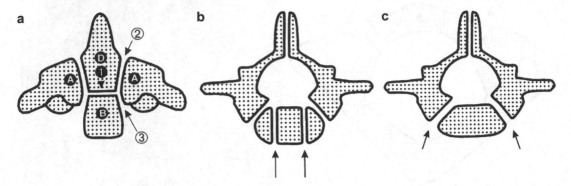

Fig. 1.7 Normal synchondroses of C2, diagrammatic representation. (**a**) Coronal plane. Note the dens (D) and body (B) of C2. Also note the synchondroses between the dens and the body (1), the dens and the neural arch (A) (2), and the body and the neural arch (3). (**b**) Axial plane. Note the parallel configuration of the synchondroses (*arrows*) between the dens and the neural arch. (**c**) Axial plane. The synchondroses (*arrows*) between the body and neural arch of C2 are more divergent

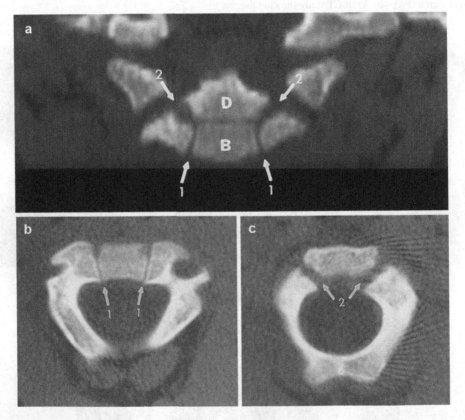

Fig. 1.8 Normal synchondroses of C2: CT demonstration. (**a**) Coronal reconstructed view. The *lower arrows* (1) identify the thin synchondroses between the body and neural arches of C2. The *upper arrows* (2) identify the wider synchondroses between the dens and the neural arch of C2. The radiolucent line between the dens (D) and body (B) of C2 represents the synchondrosis between these two structures. (**b**) Axial CT study through the body of C2 demonstrates the thin, almost parallel synchondroses between body and neural arch of C2 (1). (**c**) A slightly higher cut demonstrates the wider and more divergent synchondroses (2) between the dens and neural arch of C2

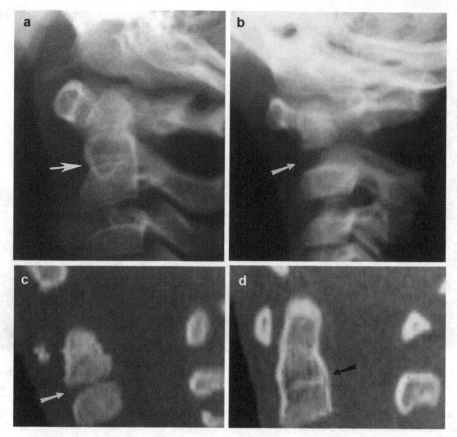

Fig. 1.9 Normal synchondrosis between the dens and the body of C2. (**a**) Note the typical radiolucent synchondrosis (*arrow*) between the dens and the body of C2. (**b**) Young infant with a very wide, and potentially confusing, but still normal synchondrosis (*arrow*) between the dens and body of C2. (**c**) Sagittal reconstructed CT image demonstrates the normal synchondrosis (*arrow*) between the dens and the body of C2 in an infant. (**d**) CT study in an older patient demonstrates virtual obliteration of the synchondrosis (*arrow*) between the dens and the body of C2

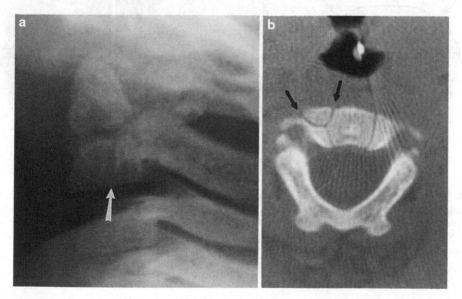

Fig. 1.10 Anomalous synchondroses of C2. (**a**) In this infant there is an anomalous synchondrosis (*arrow*) passing vertically through the body of C2. (**b**) Another patient demonstrating anomalous synchondroses of C2 (*arrows*) surrounding an isolated bony ossicle

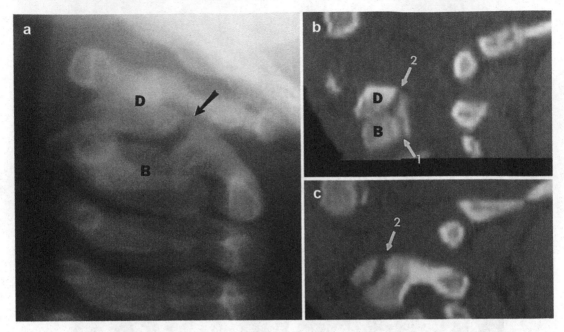

Fig. 1.11 Synchondroses of C2: Pseudofracture configurations. (**a**) Oblique view of the cervical spine demonstrates the synchondrosis (*arrow*) between neural arch and dens (D) and body (B) of C2. The horizontal radiolucent line between the dens and body represents the synchondrosis between these two structures. (**b**) Parasagittal slice on a reconstructed CT study demonstrates the pseudofracture appearance of the synchondroses between the body (B) and neural arch of C2 (1) and the dens (D) and neural arch of C2 (2). (**c**) A more lateral parasagittal CT cut demonstrates the synchondrosis between the dens and neural arch of C2 (2)

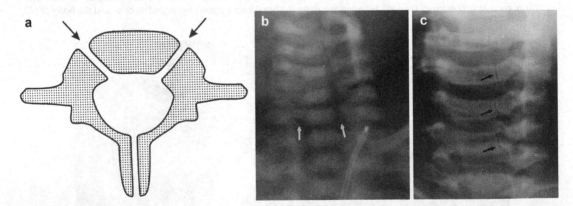

Fig. 1.12 Synchondroses of C3–C7. (**a**) Diagrammatic representation. Note the synchondroses (*arrows*) between the body and the neural arch of a typical cervical vertebral body. (**b**) Young infant, AP view of the cervical spine, demonstrates the wide defects (*arrows*) produced by the synchondroses between the body and neural arch of C2. (**c**) Older infant demonstrates the narrower appearance of the synchondroses (*arrows*) between the bodies and neural arches of the cervical vertebra as seen on this oblique view

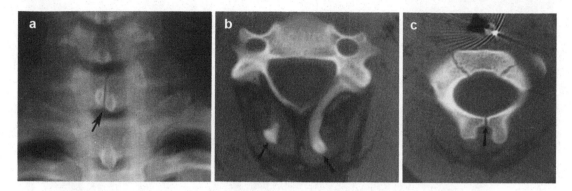

Fig. 1.13 Spina bifida occulta. (**a**) Note the spina bifida occulta (*arrow*) involving the posterior arch of C7. (**b**) In this patient note splitting of the spinous tips (*arrows*) of the neural arch of C3. (**c**) In the same patient, the second cervical vertebra demonstrates a normal posterior neural arch synchondrosis (*arrow*)

References

1. von Torklus D, Gehle W. The upper cervical spine: regional anatomy, pathology and traumatology, a systematic radiological atlas and textbook. New York: Grune & Stratton; 1972.
2. Bailey DK. The normal cervical spine in infants and children. Radiology. 1952;59:712–9.
3. Chambers AA, Gaskill MF. Midline anterior atlas clefts: CT findings. J Comput Assist Tomogr. 1992;16:868–70.
4. Swischuk LE, Hayden Jr CK, Sarwar M. The dens–arch synchondrosis versus the hangman's fracture. Pediatr Radiol. 1979;8:100–12.

Normal Variations

Vertebral Bodies and Neural Arches

In the newborn and young infant the vertebral bodies, although basically rectangular, often appear more oval because they have rounded corners, especially anteriorly (Fig. 2.1a). Thereafter the vertebral bodies become more cuboid-rectangular (Fig. 2.1b), but in some individuals can appear exceptionally flat (Fig. 2.1c). The latter configuration is not to be misinterpreted as being representative of platyspondyly, as seen with bony dysplasias, for it merely reflects the wide spectrum of the normal appearance of the vertebral bodies.

In the normal individual the neural arch of C2 usually is the largest such structure in the upper cervical spine. This is helpful when one is assessing radiographs for the presence of occipitalization. With occipitalization, C1 is fused to the base of the skull and yields to C2 as being the uppermost visualized posterior arch. Ordinarily it would be the second arch to be visualized. The posterior arch of C1 is smaller than the posterior arch of C2 and thus, when this arrangement is altered, and the uppermost visualized neural arch is the largest one present, one should suspect occipitalization.

In addition to the preceding considerations, the neural arches and spinous processes of the cervical vertebrae can show even more variation in configuration. In this regard, some may be hypoplastic, and in addition, while normal spinous processes tend to point downward, occasionally they point upward. Because of this they may erroneously suggest that a pathologic increase in the intraspinous distance is present (Fig. 2.2).

Finally, because of the complicated embryonic development of the cervico-occipital junction, aberrant bony ossicles frequently are encountered in the upper cervical spine and at the base of the skull. Most of these occur anteriorly, but they also can be seen posteriorly, and at either site usually are round or oval. Such ossicles have smooth edges and should not be misinterpreted for avulsion fractures (Fig. 2.3).

Normal Cervical Spine Motion Causing Pseudoabnormalities

In most individuals, flexion or extension of the cervical spine results in little excess motion. However, in other instances, and especially in infants and young children, since the ligaments are lax, normal physiologic hypermobility is more common and leads to spinal configurations that frequently are confused with pathologic states [1]. In addition, it is important to appreciate that the apex of the flexed cervical spine curve in infants and young children is located at a different level from that in older children and adults [2]. In infants and young children it is located in the upper cervical spine at approximately the level of C2–C3 (Fig. 2.4a), while in older children and adults it is located in the midcervical spine, that is, somewhere between C4 and C6 (Fig. 2.4b). This explains why cervical spine

L.E. Swischuk, *Imaging of the Cervical Spine in Children*, DOI 10.1007/978-1-4614-3788-8_2, © Springer Science+Business Media New York 2013

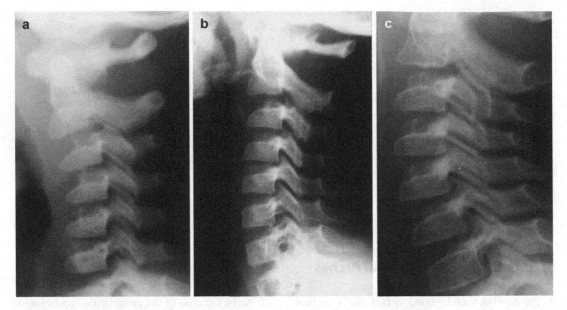

Fig. 2.1 Variable appearance of normal vertebral bodies. (a) In infancy the vertebral bodies appear more oval. (b) Typical appearance of rectangular-cuboid vertebral bodies in older children and adolescents. Note that there is some residual rounding of the upper anterior corner of C3. (c) In some patients, still normal, the vertebral bodies appear exceptionally flat

injuries, primarily flexion induced, are more common in the upper cervical spine in infants and young children, and more common at the C4–C6 level in older children, adolescents, and adults. This also is probably why degenerative changes in adults occur primarily at the C4–C6 level. In addition, when considered with the overall increased mobility of the infant's and young child's spine, it is more readily understood why so many normal hypermobility phenomena occur in the upper cervical spine in this age group.

High Anterior Arch of C1

This finding is common in young infants during hyperextension of the cervical spine [1]. The resultant configuration is that of a very high,

indeed dislocated appearing, anterior arch of C1 (Fig. 2.5). The finding, to the uninitiated can be quite alarming but, is entirely normal.

Exaggerated C1–C2 Interspinous Distance

Similar to hypermobility of the anterior arch of C1, hypermobility of C1 with flexion can result in an exaggerated intraspinous distance between C1 and C2 [1]. However, as opposed to the high anterior arch of C1 phenomenon, this configuration also can be seen in older children. Indeed, distances of up to 10 or even 12 mm can be encountered and still be normal (Fig. 2.6). In these cases, however, the C1–dens distance (predental distance) is normal.

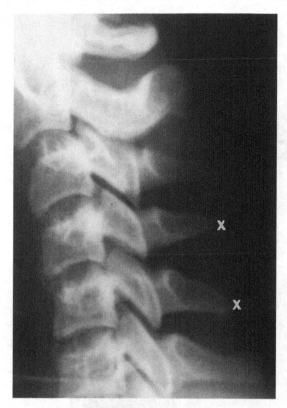

Fig. 2.2 Anomalous spinous tip configurations. Note the upward, pointing spinous tip of C4 (*upper cross symbol*). The spinous tip of C5 (X) points downward, as is more usual. However, one could misinterpret the combined findings as being representative of a flexion injury of the cervical spine, causing an increased intraspinous distance between C4 and C5

C1-to-Dens (Predental Distance)

It is well known that the predental distance in infants and young children can be wider than in adults. Indeed, up to 5 % of normal individuals can demonstrate a predental distance of 5 mm, but most often the distance is somewhere between 2 and 3 mm on initial, neutral cervical spine studies [3, 4]. In any of these cases, if there is no increase in the predental distance on flexion, the

finding can be considered normal (Fig. 2.7). However, it also should be recalled that with flexion there can be a normal increase in the distance of up to 2 mm (Fig. 2.8). If there is more widening than this, one should suspect underlying instability of the ligaments, either on a traumatic or congenital basis. The latter problem is associated with anomalies of the dens, primarily dens hypoplasia and an associated os odontoideum.

Posterior Dislocation of Vertebral Bodies

Physiologic posterior dislocation of the vertebral bodies occurs less frequently than anterior dislocation. It tends to occur over the midcervical spine, and maximum normal sliding should be no more than 2 mm [5]. The displacement can occur at one or multiple levels (Fig. 2.9).

Anterior Angulation of C2 on C3

With spasm, or rigid positioning on an "EMS transporting backboard," a patient's head can be cocked forward so that angulation of C2 on C3 results [1]. In such cases there is no actual anterior displacement of C2 on C3, but the severe degree of angulation encountered can erroneously suggest that the ligaments between C2 and C3 have been disrupted and that dislocation is present (Fig. 2.10a). In these cases I have found it helpful to draw a line along the posterior aspect of C2 and the dens and note whether it intersects or just touches the upper posterior corner of C3. If it does, no dislocation is present (Fig. 2.10b). *In such cases the posterior cervical line* [6] *should not be applied, for it will lead to erroneous conclusions.* The line was designed to be used only if anterior displacement of the body of C2 on C3 was present (see next section).

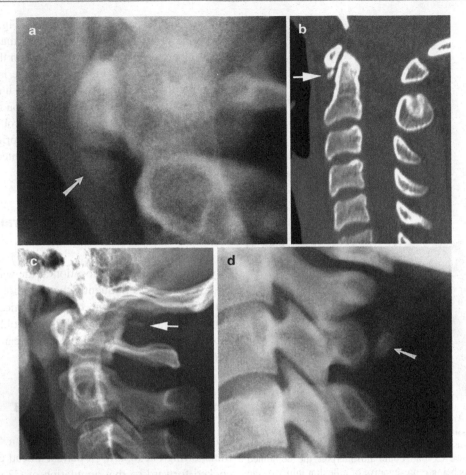

Fig. 2.3 Extra ossicles. (**a**) Note the extra ossicle (*arrow*) located below the anterior arch of C1. (**b**) In this patient, a small extra ossicle is seen along the inferior aspect of the anterior arch of C1 (*arrow*). (**c**) This patient demonstrates an extra ossicle in the posterior upper cervical region

(*arrow*). (**d**) Note the extra posterior ossicle (*arrow*) at the C3 level. Also note that the neural arch of C3 is slightly deformed and hypoplastic (i.e., smaller than the other neural arches)

Anterior Dislocation of C2 on C3

Anterior dislocation of C2 on C3 can occur with a hangman's fracture, but in infants and children it is far more common on a normal, physiologic basis [6, 7]. The degree of displacement is usually no more than 2 mm, but to the uninitiated a traumatic dislocation often is at first suggested (Fig. 2.11). In these cases I have found it helpful to apply a line, the posterior cervical line [6], to the anterior cortices of the spinous tips of C1 and C3, and then note

whether it intersects, touches, or comes close to the anterior cortex of the spinous tip of C2 (Fig. 2.12). If the line misses the anterior cortex of C2 by more than 1.5 mm, a hangman's fracture should be suspected. Otherwise, the finding should be considered physiologic (Fig. 2.13).

It is important to use the anterior cervical line only when there is anterior dislocation of C2 on C3, be it traumatic or physiologic. It has no value otherwise and will be misleading. In addition, it appears erroneously normal when there is

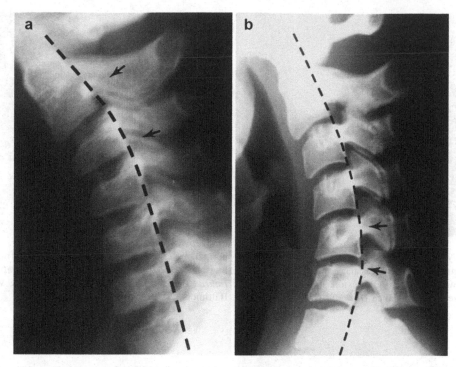

Fig. 2.4 Normal apex of flexion curve. (**a**) In infancy and young childhood, the apex of the flexion curve is at the C2–C3 level (*arrows*) (From Swischuk et al. [2].). (**b**) In older children and adolescents, the flexion curve migrates downward to a level somewhere between C4 and C6 (*arrows*)

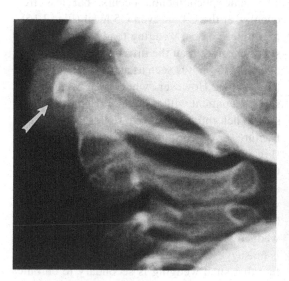

Fig. 2.5 High anterior arch of C1. With hyperextension, the normal anterior arch of C1 (*arrow*) can assume a very high location. Indeed, it may appear that the cervico-occipital junction has been disrupted

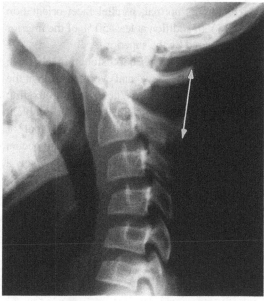

Fig. 2.6 Increased C1–C2 interspinous distance. Note the exaggerated, but normal distance (*arrowhead* to *arrowhead*) between the spinous tips of C1 and C2. Note that the predental distance is normal

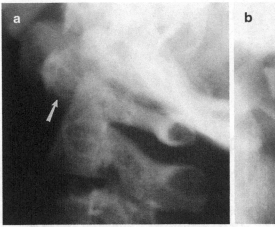 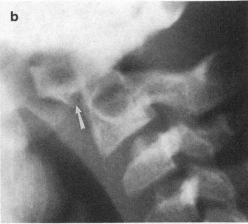

Fig. 2.7 Normal wide C1-to-dens distance. (**a**) Note the prominent C1-to-dens distance (*arrow*). The measurement was 5 mm. (**b**) On flexion, however, there is no increase in the distance (*arrow*). This patient was normal (Reproduced with permission from LE Swischuk, *Emergency Imaging of the Acutely Ill or Injured Child*, 4th ed. Lippincott Williams & Wilkins, Baltimore, 2000)

disruption of the C2–C3 apophyseal joint and ligaments without any associated fracture (i.e., no hangman's fracture). In such cases, however, the apophyseal joint appears V-shaped and abnormal while with physiologic dislocation, the apophyseal joint retains its normal, parallel facet orientation (Fig. 2.11). In addition at least 50 % of the inferior facet is covered by the superior facet.

Normal, anterior pseudodislocation also can occur at the C3–C4 level and every so often at the C4–C5 level (Fig. 2.14). When such subluxation is present at all these levels, there is no problem in identifying the configuration as normal or physiologic. It is problematic only when it occurs in isolated form, at the C2–C3 level. Once a patient reaches adolescence and young adulthood, physiologic anterior displacement of C2 on C3 tends to disappear. However, it has been documented in some young adults [8].

Wedging of C3 and C4

Anterior wedging of vertebral bodies is the hallmark of a compression fracture secondary to a hyperflexion injury. However, in the upper cervical spine of infants and young children, it is seen much more often as a normal finding [2]. In these cases physiologic hypermobility and resultant angulation of C2 on C3 lead to growth impairment of anterior upper plate of C3, producing a chronically wedged vertebra (Fig. 2.15). The same phenomenon occurs, but less frequently, at the C4, or even C5 level (Fig. 2.16). In all these cases, wedging tends to involve the superior, more than the inferior, vertebral plate, and most often it is seen as an incidental finding (Fig. 2.17). However, when such wedging is seen in a patient with trauma, it becomes necessary to determine whether it represents an acute fracture or a chronic, physiologic deformity (Fig. 2.18). This can be rapidly resolved with CT scanning: if a fracture is present, it will be apparent on the axial views. If physiologic wedging only is the problem, no fracture is seen (Fig. 2.18). In addition, on plain films the wedged vertebra has a smooth cortex and there is no suggestion of compression fracturing. The fact that such wedging is secondary to chronic compression is attested to in cases where chronic hyperflexion, due to hypotonia, can lead to the deformity (Fig. 2.19).

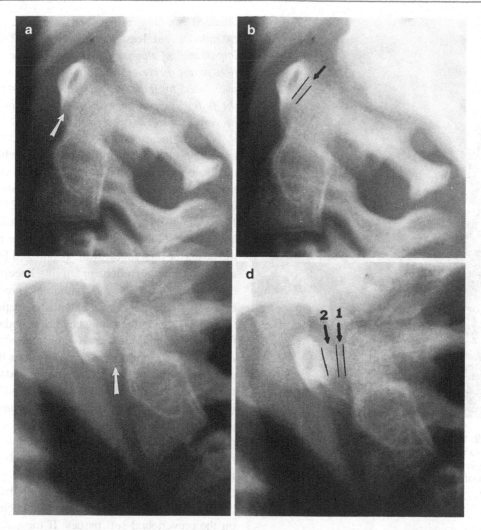

Fig. 2.8 C1-to-dens distance, maximum normal increase. (**a**) On extension, the C1-to-dens distance is normal. (**b**) The distance measures approximately 1–1.5 mm (*lines*). (**c**) On flexion, however, the predental distance increases (*arrow*). (**d**) Lines delineate the previous predental distance (1) and the new predental distance with flexion (2). Overall, the increase in distance with flexion is no more than 2 mm. Also note that the predental distance normally is slightly wider superiorly

Physiologic wedging gradually disappears as the individual gets older and the apex of the flexed cervical spine shifts downward to the midcervical level. As this happens, the chronic compressive forces on C3, and C4, are removed and the vertebrae are allowed to grow back to their original configuration. This probably is why the deformity is not seen in older children, adolescents, or adults.

Normal Apophyseal Joints: Older Child

Because the flexion curve in older children and adolescents is in the lower cervical spine, some patients demonstrate slight hypermobility through the apophyseal joints in this area (Fig. 2.20). As a result joints may appear slightly V-shaped, but on flexion there will be

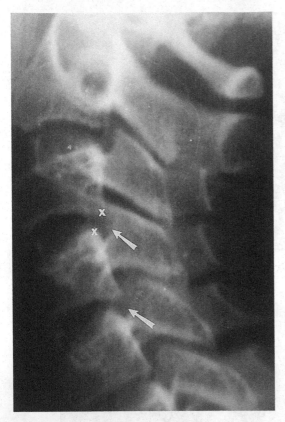

Fig. 2.9 Normal posterior displacement of vertebral bodies (*cross symbols*). Note posterior displacement of C3 on C4 (*upper arrow*) and less, but still present, posterior displacement of C4 on C5 (*lower arrow*). This patient was normal

no excessive motion. This configuration is acceptable as a normal variation in older children and adolescents (Fig. 2.20).

Prevertebral Soft Tissues

The prevertebral soft tissues are notoriously difficult to evaluate in infants and young children. Mostly this is because of buckling of the airway on expiration and poor (neck is flexed) positioning (Fig. 2.21). To properly evaluate the prevertebral soft tissues, the study should be obtained on inspiration and with the neck extended or at least straight (Fig. 2.22). *The importance of this particular aspect of evaluation of the prevertebral soft tissues cannot be overstated, for if the study is improperly obtained, the initial impression will be that of pathologic prevertebral soft tissue thickening.*

Normal measurements are available, but I have found it more useful to determine whether the posterior pharyngeal wall is located posterior to the posterior tracheal wall. This results in a stepoff of the air column at this level (Figs. 2.22b, c). If this stepoff is present, the prevertebral soft tissues likely are normal [1]. If, on the other hand, the posterior pharyngeal wall, as outlined by air, is in a continuous straight, or curving lineup with the posterior tracheal wall, pathologic prevertebral soft tissue thickening should be suspected (Fig. 2.23). Such thickening can be secondary to trauma (hematoma), abscess, lymph node enlargement, a variety of tumors, myxedematous thickening in cretinism [9], and edema secondary to the superior vena cava syndrome [10]. In addition it might be noted that the normally prominent prevertebral tissues just anterior to C1 and C2 now can be clearly demonstrated with magnetic resonance (MR) techniques and even can be seen in older children (Fig. 2.24).

Finally over the years I have come to the conclusion that one should not spend too much time on the prevertebral soft tissues. If they tell you something immediately then use them, if they do not, go on to something else.

Ring Epiphysis

All vertebral bodies have ring epiphyses over their superior and inferior plates. On lateral view these epiphyses appear as triangular or sliver-like bony fragments (Fig. 2.25a). They should not be confused with corner avulsion fractures. However, it should be noted that the ring epiphysis can be avulsed in children and present as a form of the teardrop fracture [11].

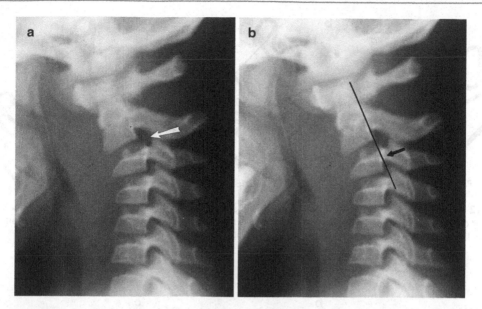

Fig. 2.10 Anterior angulation of C2 on C3. (**a**) Note that C2 is angled forward on C3 (*arrow*). (**b**) However, the line drawn along the posterior aspect of C2 does not intersect C3, but just touches the upper posterior corner of C3 (*arrow*). Therefore, there is no anterior dislocation. However, the prominent, but normal, C1-to-dens distance, generous C1–C2 interspinous distance, along with thickening of the soft tissues, due to improper technique, could lead one to erroneously diagnose a severe hyperflexion injury of the upper cervical spine

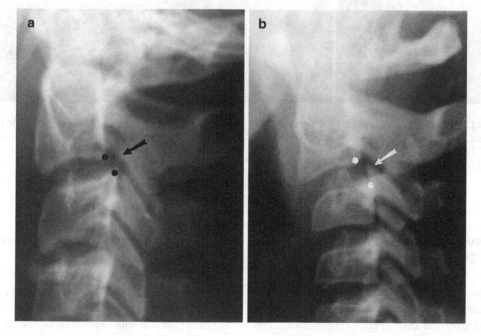

Fig. 2.11 Physiologic anterior subluxation of C2 on C3. (**a**) Note that C2 is anteriorly displaced on C3 (*dots* and *arrow*). (**b**) Another patient with similar findings (*dots* and *arrow*). Note that the apophyseal joint facets are parallel

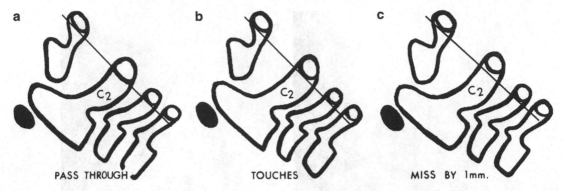

Fig. 2.12 Posterior cervical line: normal limits. (**a**) The posterior cervical line touches the anterior cortex of C2. (**b**) The line passes through the anterior cortex of the spinous tip of C2. (**c**) The posterior cervical line misses the anterior cortex of C2 by only 1 mm (From Cattell and Filtzer [7])

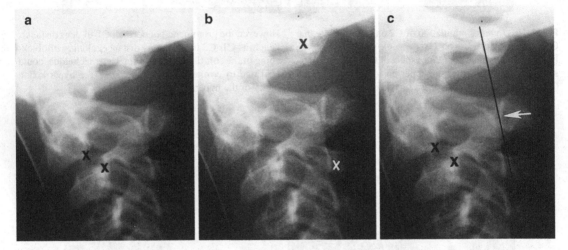

Fig. 2.13 Physiologic subluxation C2–C3 posterior cervical line. (**a**) There is marked anterior displacement of C2 on C3 (*cross symbols*). (**b**) *Cross symbols* delineate the locations of the cortices of C1 and C3 for drawing of the posterior cervical line. (**c**) The *arrow* points to the posterior cervical line drawn from the anterior cortex of C1 to the anterior cortex of C3 which passes through the anterior cortex of C2. It is normal

Transverse Process Projection Over Disk Spaces

The transverse processes of the vertebrae can be projected, with slight obliquity, so that they are viewed over the disk spaces (Fig. 2.25b). This finding should not be misinterpreted for an avulsion or compression fracture of a vertebral body.

Pseudowidening of the Spinal Canal

In infants, it is very common for the spinal canal, on anteroposterior (AP) view, to appear to be pathologically widened (Fig. 2.25c). This phenomenon can be exaggerated with slight obliquity of the spine (Fig. 2.25d), but it is entirely normal and is not a problem on lateral views of the cervical spine.

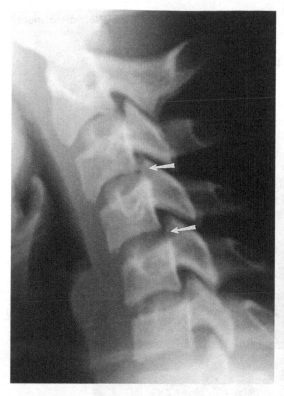

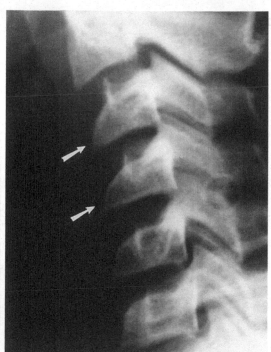

Fig. 2.16 Normal wedged vertebra: multiple levels. Note anterior wedging of both C3 and C4 (*arrows*)

Fig. 2.14 Multiple physiologic anterior subluxations. Note that C3 is anteriorly displaced on C4 (*upper arrow*) and that C4 is anteriorly displaced on C5 (*lower arrow*)

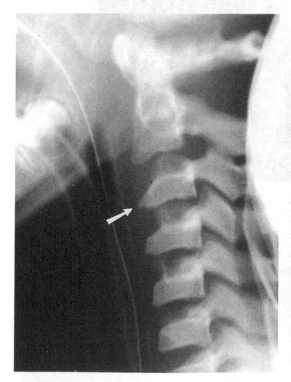

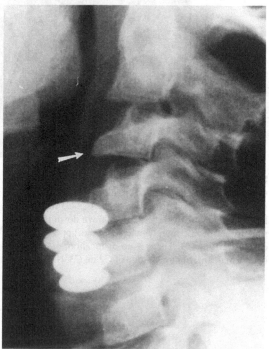

Fig. 2.15 Normal anterior wedging of C3. Note the wedged appearance (*arrow*) of C3. Also note that the deformity involves the superior plate more than the inferior plate. The prevertebral soft tissues are somewhat prominent in this patient, but the patient was normal

Fig. 2.17 Wedging of C3: incidental finding. Note the wedged appearance of C3 (*arrow*). Again note that the superior plate is almost exclusively involved in producing the wedging configuration. This patient had no cervical spine trauma

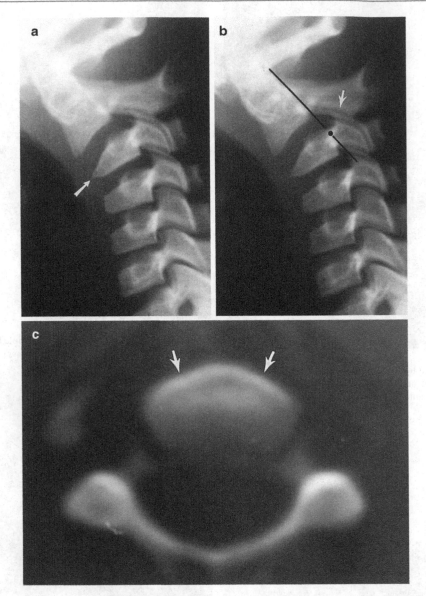

Fig. 2.18 Anterior wedging of C3 with pseudodisloca-tion appearance of spine. (**a**) Note the pronounced wedg-ing of C3 (*arrow*). Dislocation at the C2–C3 level might be suggested. (**b**) However, a line drawn down the poste-rior aspect of C2 merely intersects the upper posterior corner (*dot*) of C3. There is no dislocation, only severe, but normal, anterior angulation of C2 on C3. Note that the apophyseal joint (*arrow*) is normal in that the facets are parallel. The appearance of 50 % coverage of the facet is normal. (**c**) CT study demonstrates no fracture of the body of C3 (*arrows*) ((**a**, **c**) Reproduced with permission from LE Swischuk, *Emergency Radiology of the Acutely Ill or Injured Child*, 4th ed. Lippincott Williams & Wilkins, Baltimore, 2000)

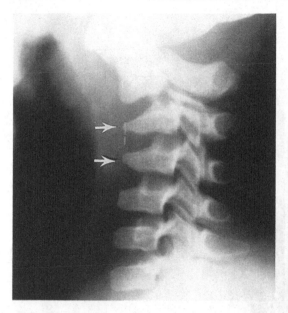

Fig. 2.19 Chronic wedging, no trauma. Note severe wedging of multiple vertebrae in this patient with chronic hypotonia (*arrows*)

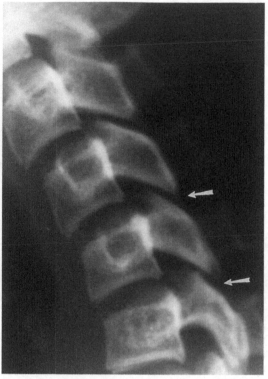

Fig. 2.20 Lower cervical apophyseal joints. Note the slight V-shaped configuration of at least two of the lower cervical apophyseal joints (*arrows*). There was no excessive motion at these sites, and this degree of V-shaped configuration can be considered physiologic and normal in older children and adolescents

Positioning Pseudofractures of the Upper Cervical Spine

With obliquity and slight rotation, the posterior arches of C1–C3 can appear to be fractured or offset and overall, alarmingly abnormal (Fig. 2.26a–c). In addition, with slight lateral tilting of the head and neck, the cortices of the posterior arch of C2 can become offset, erroneously suggesting an avulsion fracture (Fig. 2.26d).

Bilateral Offset Lateral Masses of C1 (Increase in Dens–Lateral Mass Distance)

Laterally offset masses of C1 on C2 are characteristic of Jefferson compression fractures of C1. However, under the age of 2 years, because of a differential growth factor, the lateral masses of C1 can normally appear to be offset [12]. This is important to appreciate, for the finding can be misinterpreted for traumatic lateral displacement of the lateral masses (Fig. 2.27).

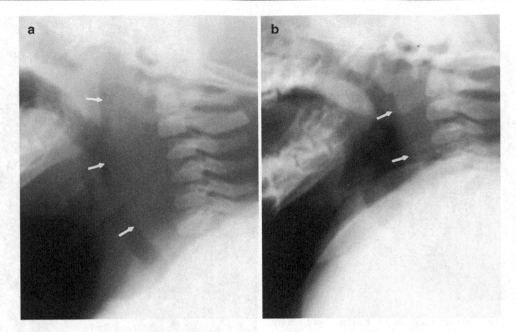

Fig. 2.21 Pseudoprominent prevertebral soft tissues. (**a**) In this patient the prevertebral soft tissues appear alarmingly wide. Indeed, the posterior wall of the pharynx and trachea almost forms a continuous arc (*arrows*). (**b**) With deep inspiration, however, the hypopharynx distends with air and the posterior pharyngeal wall now is in its normal posterior location. The slight remaining degree of prevertebral soft tissue prominence is normal in infancy

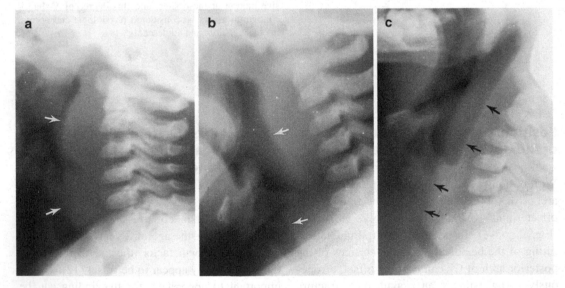

Fig. 2.22 Pseudoprevertebral soft tissue thickening: various phases. (**a**) Note the bilobed appearance of the apparently thickened prevertebral soft tissues (*arrows*). (**b**) With slightly deeper inspiration, the posterior wall of the hypopharynx (*upper arrow*) is more clearly delineated. It is located posterior to the air column of the trachea (*lower arrow*). (**c**) With full inspiration, the normal stepoff (*arrows*) between the posterior hypopharyngeal wall and posterior tracheal wall is clearly apparent

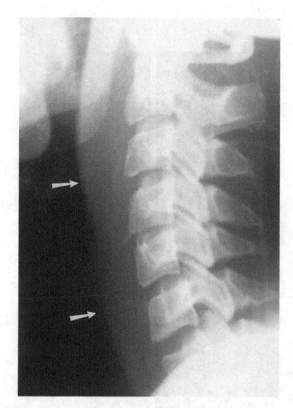

Fig. 2.23 Pathologic prevertebral soft tissue thickening. Note the continuous arc formed by the posterior wall of the hypopharynx (*upper arrow*) and the posterior wall of the upper trachea (*lower arrow*). There is a small teardrop fracture involving C5. The disk space between C4 and C5 also is narrowed. All these findings indicate the presence of an underlying flexion injury at this level

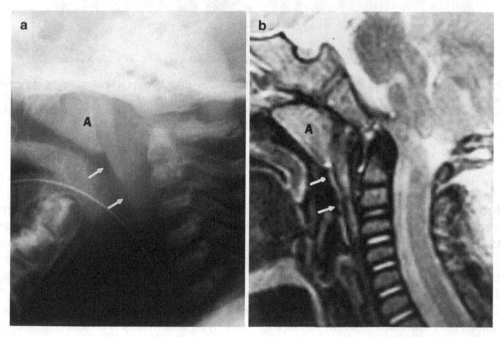

Fig. 2.24 Prominent adenoids and prevertebral soft tissues. (**a**) The adenoids (A) are prominent and the upper prevertebral soft tissues appear alarmingly wide (*arrow*). (**b**) Magnetic resonance imaging demonstrated the prominent adenoids (A) and prevertebral soft tissues (*arrows*). This patient had no trauma

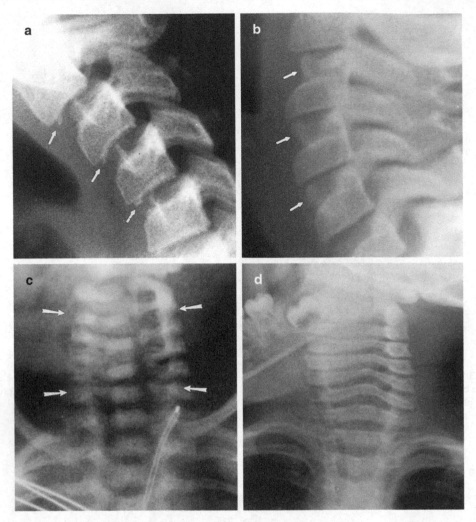

Fig. 2.25 (a) Normal "ring" epiphysis. Note the bony, fragment-like appearance (*arrows*) of the normal ring epiphysis. (b) Normal transverse processes. With slight rotation, the transverse processes (*arrows*), can be projected through the disk spaces. (c) Pseudowidening of the cervical spinal canal (*arrows*). Note the wide appearance of the spinal canal. (d) Rotation leads to exaggerated pseudowidening of the cervical spinal canal

Unilateral Offset Lateral Mass of C1 (Increased Unilateral Dens–Lateral Mass Distance)

Most often unilateral offsetting of the lateral mass of C1 is secondary to rotation. *In these cases the lateral mass–dens distance is increased on one side, but on the contralateral side the distance is narrower than normal* (Fig. 2.28). Such normal rotation-induced discrepancies in the distance from dens to lateral mass now are commonly seen on CT studies [13]. Finally, it should be noted that in children, hypermobility of the upper cervical spine can lead to significant lateral displacement of the lateral masses of C1 and yet no underlying abnormality is present (Fig. 2.29).

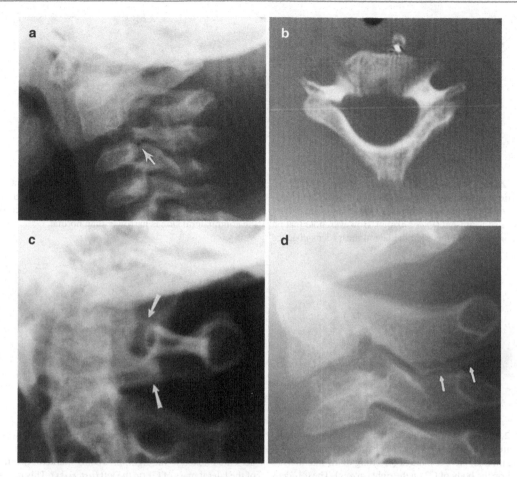

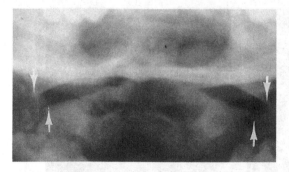

Fig. 2.26 Pseudofractures. (**a**) With rotation, the posterior arch of C3 appears to be separated and dislocated from the body of C3 (*arrow*). (**b**) CT study demonstrates that no fractures are present. (**c**) In this patient, with rotation, unilateral posterior C1 arch fracture–dislocation is erroneously suggested (*arrow*). (**d**) Slight rotation produces offsetting of the posterior limbs of the neural arch of C2, leading to an avulsion fracture-like appearance (*arrows*)

Fig. 2.27 Pseudo-offsetting; lateral masses of C1 in infancy. Note apparent bilateral offsetting of the lateral masses of C1 on C2 (*arrows*). In infancy, this pseudo-Jefferson fracture appearance is normal (Reproduced with permission from LE Swischuk, *Emergency Radiology of the Acutely Ill or Injured Child*, 4th ed. Lippincott Williams & Wilkins, Baltimore, 2000)

Central Veins

The central veins of the vertebral bodies often can be misinterpreted for fractures. This is important to appreciate, especially in the absence of other evidence of trauma to the vertebral body (Fig. 2.30).

Posticus Ponticus

The posticus ponticus represents a partial or complete bony encirclement of the vertebral artery as it exits the spinal canal and enters the calvarium. Usually there is no problem in identifying this structure (Fig. 2.31).

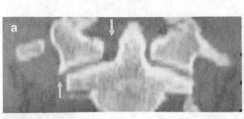

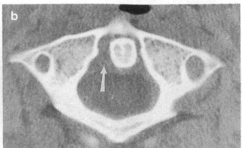

Fig. 2.28 Pseudo-offsetting lateral mass of C1. (**a**) Rotation causes widening of the lateral mass–dens distance on the right (*upper arrow*). Offsetting of the lateral mass also is present (*lower arrow*). However, note that on the contralateral other side the lateral mass–dens distance is narrower than normal. (**b**) Axial CT of the same patient demonstrates slight rotation and increase in the right lateral mass–dens distance (*arrow*). The same distance on the contralateral side is narrower than normal

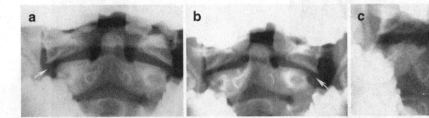

Fig. 2.29 Hypermobility of C1 on C2, pseudopathologic offsetting. (**a**) In this patient, who sustained mild cervical spine trauma, there is marked offsetting of the lateral mass of C1 on the body of C2 on the right (*arrow*). The C1–dens distance also is increased. (**b**) Just a few moments later, it is the left lateral mass that appears to be offset (*arrow*) on the body of C2. (**c**) Under fluoroscopic control, the patient's neck was flexed to the right, producing marked offsetting of the lateral mass of C1 on the left (*asterisks*). This patient had no pain and no limitation of motion. He was normal

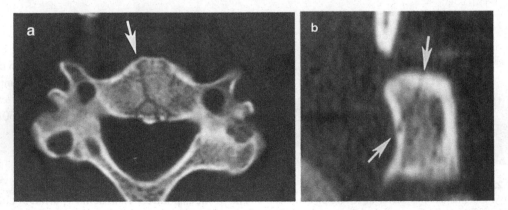

Fig. 2.30 Central vein and course trabeculae pseudofractures. (**a**) Note the stellate appearance of the central veins (*arrows*). (**b**) Sagittal reconstructed view demonstrates a similar pseudofracture appearance (*arrows*). (**c**) In this patient a fracture is suggested through the neural arch (*arrow*) because of the confluence of a venous groove and trabecular markings. (**d**) Sagittal reconstructed view demonstrates no fracture (*arrow*) at the site

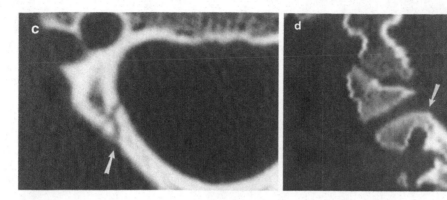

Fig. 2.30 (continued)

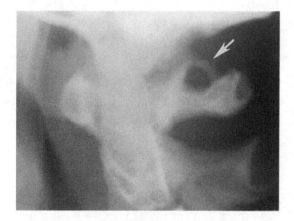

Fig. 2.31 Posticus ponticus. Note the typical appearance of the posticus ponticus (*arrow*)

References

1. Swischuk LE. Normal cervical spine variations mimicking injuries in children. Emerg Radiol. 1999; 6:299–306.
2. Swischuk LE, Swischuk PN, John SD. Wedging of C-3 in infants and children: usually a normal finding and not a fracture. Radiology. 1993;188:523–6.
3. Locke GR, Gardner JI, Van Epps EF. Atlas–dens interval (ADI) in children: a survey based on 200 normal cervical spines. Am J Roentgenol Radium Ther Nucl Med. 1996;97:135–40.
4. Swischuk LE. Emergency radiology of the acutely ill or injured child. 3rd ed. Baltimore: Williams & Wilkins; 1994. p. 659.
5. Clark WM, Gehweiler Jr JA, Laib R. Twelve significant signs of cervical spine trauma. Skeletal Radiol. 1979;3:2201–5.
6. Swischuk LE. Anterior displacement of C2 in children: physiologic or pathologic? A helpful differentiating line. Radiology. 1977;122:759–63.
7. Cattell HS, Filtzer DL. Pseudosubluxation and other normal variations in the cervical spine in children. J Bone Joint Surg Am. 1965;47A:1295–309.
8. Harrison RB, Keats TE, Winn HR, Riddervold HO, Pope Jr TL. Pseudosubluxation in the axis in young adults. J Can Assoc Radiol. 1980;31:176–7.
9. Grunebaum M, Moskowitz G. The retropharyngeal soft tissues in young infants with hypothyroidism. Am J Roentgenol Radium Ther Nucl Med. 1970;108:543–5.
10. Swischuk LE, Crowe JE, Mewborne Jr EB. Large vein of Galen aneurysms in the neonate: a constellation of diagnostic chest and neck radiologic findings. Pediatr Radiol. 1977;6:4–9.
11. Gooding CA, Hurwitz ME. Avulsed vertebral rim apophysis in a child. Pediatr Radiol. 1974;2:265–8.
12. Suss RA, Zimmerman RD, Leeds NE. Pseudospread of the atlas: false sign of Jefferson fracture in young children. AJR Am J Roentgenol. 1983;140:1079–82.
13. Wolansky LJ, Rajaraman V, Seo C, et al. The lateral atlanto–dens interval: normal range of asymmetry. Emerg Radiol. 1999;6:290–3.

Fig. 2. ...

References

Anomalies

3

Fusion–Segmentation Anomalies

Occurring alone or as part of some syndrome, fusion–segmentation anomalies range from hemivertebra through cleft vertebrae to absence of a vertebral body. The embryology of these anomalies is presented in Chap. 1 (Figs. 1.2 and 1.3).

Midline vertebral body clefts usually are of no serious clinical consequence and are manifest primarily as butterfly or cleft vertebrae (Fig. 3.1). Most often no associated problem exists, but occasionally one can encounter such vertebrae with neurenteric or enteric duplication cysts. Sagittal hemivertebrae usually are associated with focal scoliosis (see later: Fig. 3.8). Coronal cleft and coronal hemivertebrae are less common, but the latter, especially when the anterior half of the vertebra is missing, can lead to spine instability (Fig. 3.2a, b). Finally, the entire vertebral body or bodies may be hypoplastic or absent [1], and again instability usually is present (Fig. 3.2c). Coronally cleft vertebrae are more common in the thoracolumbar spine, can be seen in syndromes such as trisomy 13–15 and rhizomelic punctate epiphyseal dysplasia and also are more common in males than in females [2]. They are, however, uncommonly encountered in the cervical spine.

Fusion Anomalies of Vertebral Bodies

Fusion anomalies most commonly occur at the C2–C3 level, and such fusion frequently involves the associated apophyseal joints (Fig. 3.3). Fusion also can occur at lower levels and may be multiple (Fig. 3.4). In all these cases, the intervening disk may be completely obliterated or variably narrowed (Fig. 3.4). In addition, the involved vertebral bodies tend to taper toward the rudimentary disk (Fig. 3.4); interestingly, the disks above and below the level of fusion often are enlarged or hypertrophied. This is important to appreciate, for unless cord compression is seen these hypertrophied disks should not be interpreted as representing pathologic degeneration and herniation. This manifestation of vertebral fusion is best demonstrated with MRI (Fig. 3.5).

C1 and C2 also can fuse, and often such fusion is associated with anomalous dens development (Fig. 3.6). This is important because while most cases of fusion at lower levels are not a clinical problem, this is not always true in the upper cervical spine: In the upper cervical spine, when there is enough associated anomalous formation, instability can be present (Fig. 3.7).

When fusion anomalies are extensive, and accompanied by segmentation (hemivertebra) anomalies, bizarre configurations are common.

L.E. Swischuk, *Imaging of the Cervical Spine in Children*,
DOI 10.1007/978-1-4614-3788-8_3, © Springer Science+Business Media New York 2013

This most commonly occurs in the Klippel–Feil syndrome, but interestingly, even if the cervical spine appears very bizarre and distorted (Fig. 3.8), only seldom is neurologic deficit a problem.

However, these patients also can have associated congenital deafness, renal anomalies, and Sprengel's deformity (Fig. 3.9) of the scapula [3–5]. Neurologic deficit is more likely to occur in adulthood, and finally a rare form of severe fusion–segmentation abnormality occurs in usually lethal iniencephaly [6], a condition in which the underdeveloped upper cervical spine is fused to the occiput (Fig. 3.10).

Fusion of C1 to the base of the skull constitutes so-called *occipitalization*, and fusion can be complete, partial, unilateral, and either bony or fibrous (Fig. 3.11). In any of these cases, the uppermost neural arch is the largest one visible and thus should be the posterior arch of C2 (Fig. 3.11). Therefore, even though one does not come to the conclusion on initial inspection that C1 is fused with the base of the skull, the presence of this large uppermost neural arch and spinous process should provide the proper clue to the underlying diagnosis. Suspected occipitalization is easily confirmed with flexion views and CT

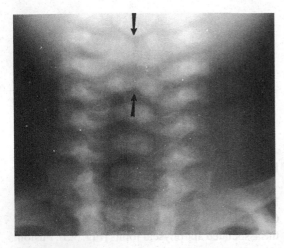

Fig. 3.1 Butterfly vertebra. Note central vertebral body narrowing (*arrows*), resulting in a butterfly vertebra

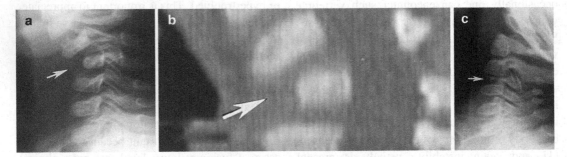

Fig. 3.2 Coronal segmentation anomalies and absent vertebrae. (**a**) Coronal hemivertebra. The anterior portion of the fourth cervical vertebra did not develop, resulting in a small vertebral body (coronal hemivertebra) and marked kyphosis at the C3–C4 level (*arrow*). (**b**) Sagittal reconstructed CT study demonstrates similar findings (*arrow*). (**c**) Absent vertebral body. In this patient the entire vertebral body of C3 is markedly underdeveloped and virtually absent (*arrow*). In addition, while the pedicles are developed, the posterior neural arch is not. Posterior neural arch underdevelopment also is present at the C4 and C5 levels

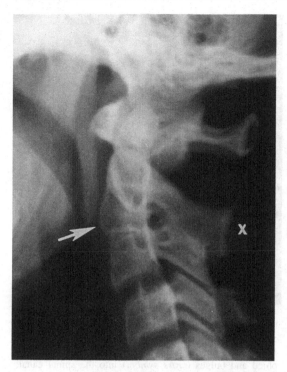

Fig. 3.3 Fusion C2–C3. Note fusion of the vertebral bodies of C2 and C3 (*arrow*). Fusion extends to the posterior elements; the neural arches and the spinous processes. There is only one spinous tip (*cross symbol*) for both C2 and C3

of the cervical spine where the fused posterior arch of C1 is easier to assess (Fig. 3.12).

The more severe the abnormality, the more likelihood of clinical problems as the dens protrudes more and more into the foramen magnum (basilar invagination) and encroaches on the brain stem (Fig. 3.13). When basilar invagination of the dens is present, there often is associated platybasia of the skull. Occipitalization also can be associated with vertebral fusions at other levels in the cervical spine, and basilar invagination can be acquired when the skull base is underossified or softened. This can occur with osteogenesis imperfecta and metabolic bone conditions leading to undermineralization of the skull.

Posterior C1 Arch Defects

Fibrous posterior C1 arch defects can appear very bizarre, for often there is marked hypoplasia of the neural arch, but in other cases only a small defect occurs (Fig. 3.14). The ends of the bones involved in any of these cases show smooth, well-corticated margins, and the bony remnants

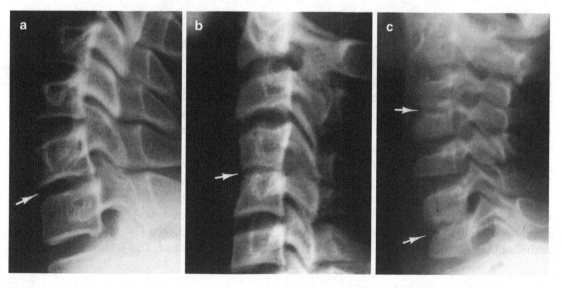

Fig. 3.4 Vertebral fusion: lower cervical spine. (**a**) Note the slightly narrowed intervertebral disk (*arrow*) between C6 and C7. (**b**) The disk (*arrow*) between the fused C4 and C5 cervical vertebrae is very narrow. Also note that the involved vertebrae are smaller than normal and taper toward the narrowed disk. (**c**) Fusions are present at both the C3–C4 and C6–C7 levels (*arrows*). The disk spaces are narrowed and almost obliterated. C3 and C4 are smaller than normal

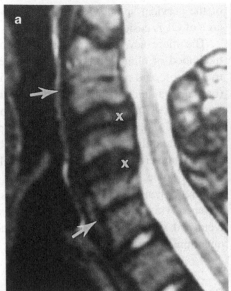 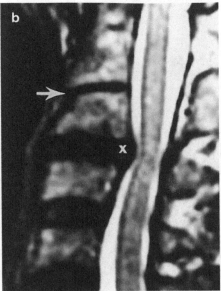

Fig. 3.5 Vertebral fusion with hypertrophied interverte- bral disks. (**a**) In this patient two levels of fusion (nar- rowed disks) are present (*arrows*). The large, hypertrophied intervening disks (*cross symbols*) bulge into the spinal canal but do not encroach upon the spinal cord. Note that the involved disks also have lost their normal high signal on this T2-weighted image. (**b**) In this patient there is fusion of C2 and C3 (*arrow*). The disk below is hypertro- phied and bulges (*cross symbol*) into the spinal canal, causing slight compression of the spinal cord

may be triangular or tapered. In some instances the defect is very large, while in others one side, or the entire bony neural arch, is absent. All these anomalies are readily demonstrable with plain films and CT studies (Fig. 3.15), but it should be underscored that unless there is associated, significant hypoplasia of the dens, the anomaly is stable (Fig. 3.16). On the other hand, if dens hypoplasia coexists, instability becomes a problem and is discussed in more detail in the Chap. 4. In the meantime, the upper cervical spine is very subject to congenital anomalies and at times bizarre configurations result (Fig. 3.17).

Posterior C2 Arch Defects

Although less common than defects of C1, posterior C2 arch defects often are more prob- lematic. The reason for this is that they must be differentiated from a hangman's fracture. A hang- man's fracture represents an unstable injury and interestingly enough is not uncommon in infancy. However, in terms of differentiating the two problems, if the bony defect of C2 is congenital in origin, the entire neural arch usually is under- developed or elongated [7–11], and the edges of the defect are smooth and sclerotic (Fig. 3.18).

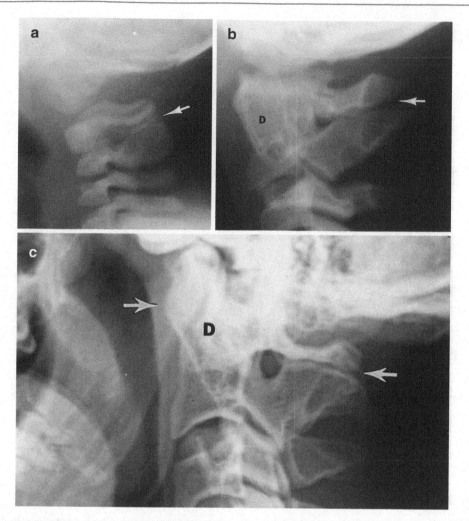

Fig. 3.6 C1–C2 fusion. (**a**) Note fusion of the posterior arches of C1 and C2 (*arrow*). (**b**) Older child demonstrating posterior fusion of C1 and C2 (*arrow*). The dens (D) is deformed, and there is no ossification of the anterior arch of C1. (**c**) In this patient there is anomalous formation of the fused neural arches of C1 and C2 (*posterior arrow*). The anterior arch of C1 is hypertrophied (*anterior arrow*) and the dens (D) is underdeveloped. The cervical spine in all these patients was stable

In addition, in some cases the neural arch of C2 is somewhat dysplastic (Fig. 3.19). This is an important point to note, for with hangman's fractures, the neural arch of C2 appears normal. In all of these cases however, the fact that the defect is stable on flexion is most important for if it is unstable, and widens on flexion, it most likely represents a hangman's fracture. In spite of this, there often is considerable difference of opinion and discussion about this matter. To this end, Guararino [12] has suggested that a spectrum of abnormality exists, identifying three types of defect: (1) a congenital defect with no abnormal motion, (2) an acquired traumatic spondyloysis

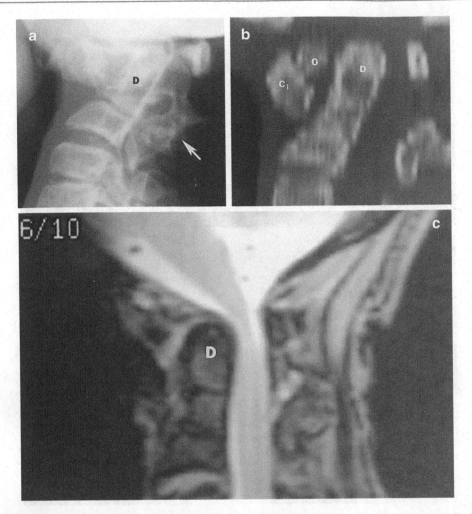

Fig. 3.7 Fusion: upper cervical spine with instability. (**a**) Note marked deformity and fusion of the posterior elements of C2 and C3 (*arrow*). The dens (D) is posteriorly tilted and slightly underdeveloped. The predental distance is increased. (**b**) Sagittal reconstructed CT study demonstrates the posteriorly tilted dens (D); here the wide predental distance seen in (**a**) is filled with a displaced os odontoideum (O). The anterior arch of C1 (C₁) is deformed and overgrown. (**c**) Sagittal MR study demonstrates that the dens (D) is encroaching upon the spinal canal and causing compression of the upper cord

with abnormal motion, and (3) a frank hangman's fracture. The latter two however, probably represent the same entity. All this is especially important in infants where hangman's fractures often are considered rare. However, these fractures are being recognized more frequently [13–16], and in the past, many probably were misinterpreted as congenital defects. To further complicate matters, these fractures can be relatively silent clinically [16]. In the end, whatever etiologic approach one takes, if on flexion the defect widens, it requires surgical stabilization.

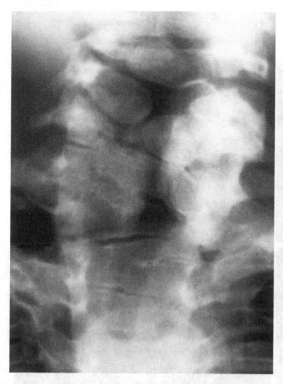

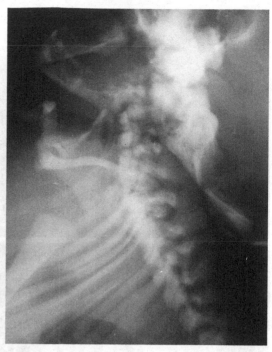

Fig. 3.8 Klippel–Feil syndrome. Note extensive fusion–segmentation anomalies of the entire cervical spine

Fig. 3.10 Iniencephaly. (**a**) Note the underdeveloped, malformed cervical spine, which basically is fused with the occiput. The patient's neck is held in extreme extension (Reproduced with permission from LE Swischuk, *Imaging of the Newborn Infant and Young Child*, Lippincott Williams & Wilkins, Baltimore, 1997)

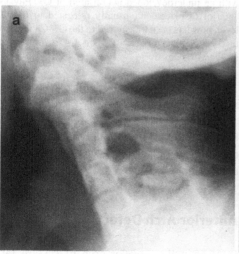

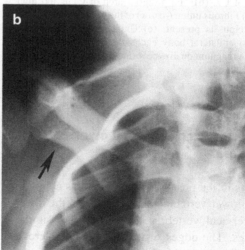

Fig. 3.9 Klippel–Feil syndrome with Sprengel's deformity. (**a**) Note extensive fusion–segmentation anomalies through both the vertebral bodies and posterior arches of the cervical spine. (**b**) Same patient. The right scapula is rotated and elevated (*arrow*), constituting Sprengel's deformity

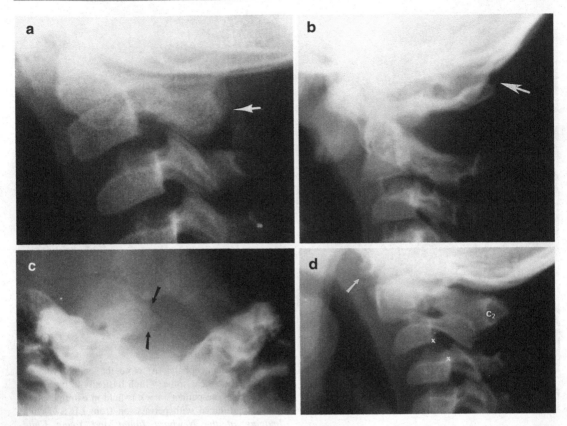

Fig. 3.11 Occipitalization: various configurations. (**a**) Note that the anterior and posterior arches of C1 are not visible because they are fused with the base of the skull. The uppermost spinous tip (*arrow*) is the largest visualized. It is that of C2. (**b**) The posterior arch of C1 is too high (*arrow*) Fibrous union (*arrow*) of the posterior arch of C1 and occiput is present. (**c**) Unilateral occipitalization leads to unilateral bony encroachment (*arrows*) of the foramen magnum on Towne's view. (**d**) In this patient the anterior arch of C1 (*arrow*) is small and fused to the base of the skull. The posterior arch, which has been incorporated into the base of the skull, is not visible. The uppermost spinous process is that of C2 (C_2), and it is fused with an underdeveloped neural arch of C3. Physiologic anterior displacement, usually relegated to the C2–C3 level, now has been transferred to the C3–C4 level, where marked displacement of C3 on C4 is present (*cross symbols*)

Posterior Arch Defects: Lower Vertebra

Defects in the posterior arch are not as common in the lower vertebrae as those seen in the upper two cervical vertebrae, but they show similar findings. The edges of the defects are sclerotic and well corticated [17–19]. If such defects occur at a single level, they usually are stable (Fig. 3.20). However, if they occur at multiple levels the spine becomes unstable. In any case, one usually proceed to flexion extension views, possibly CT, but more likely MR with flexion and extension to determine whether there was any instability or cord compression.

Anterior Arch Defects of C1

Defects in the anterior arch of C1 are far less common than are those in the posterior C1 arch. In addition, despite the anterior arch of C1 being quite hypoplastic, the entire configuration is stable (Fig. 3.21).

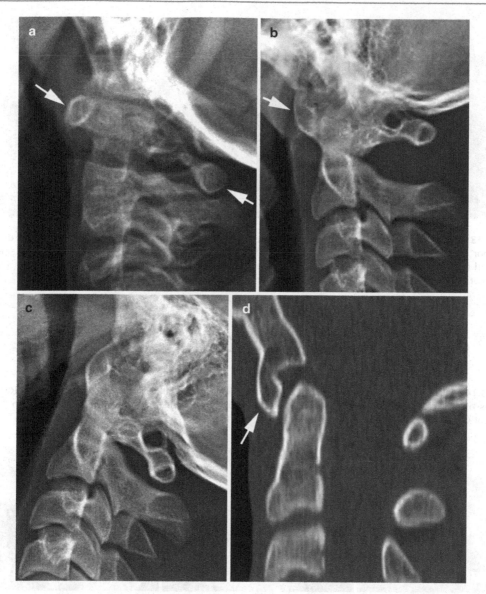

Fig. 3.12 Occipitalization of C1: other configurations (**a**) C1 is dysplastic (*arrows*). In addition it is closely adherent to the occiput because of fibrous union. (**b**) Another patient. The anterior arch of C1 is closely apposed to the calvarium (*arrows*). The neural arch is in close proximity to the occiput. (**c**) With extension there is no change in position of the posterior arch of C1. It is fused to the occiput by fibrous tissue. (**d**) Sagittal CT study demonstrates the close position of the spinous tip of C1 to the occiput and that the anterior arch of C1 (*arrow*) is fused with the occiput

Dysplastic Neural Arches

When only one neural arch is dysplastic, the anomaly usually is of no particular consequence. However, when multiple neural arches are involved [20, 21], the spine can become unstable (Fig. 3.22). Neural arch dysplasia can occur on an isolated basis but also is commonly seen with neurofibromatosis.

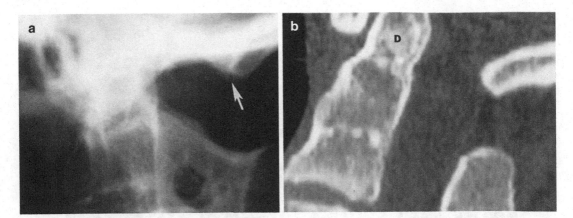

Fig. 3.13 Basilar invagination. (**a**) In this patient the posterior arch of C1 is small and fused to the base of the skull (*arrow*). The anterior arch is not visible. The dens, not clearly visible, protrudes into the foramen magnum. (**b**) Sagittal reconstructed CT study demonstrates the high position of the dens (D) invaginating into the foramen magnum, constituting basilar invagination

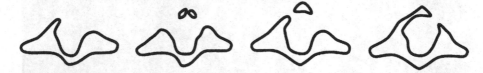

Fig. 3.14 Diagrammatic representation of various degrees of posterior C1 arch defects. Note the various posterior C1 arch defects (Modified from von Torklus D, Gehle W. The Upper Cervical Spine: Regional Morphology, Pathology, and Traumatology; An X-Ray Atlas. New York: Grune & Stratton; 1972)

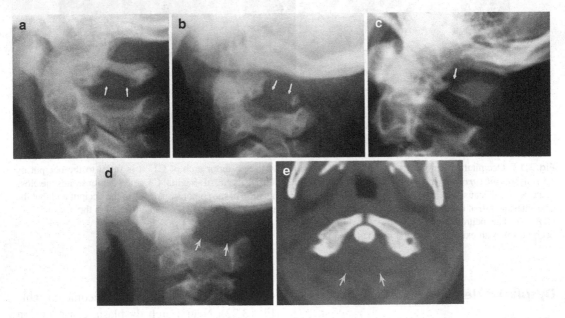

Fig. 3.15 C1 posterior arch underdevelopment and defects. (**a**) Unilateral absence (*arrows*) of the posterior arch of C1. (**b**) A large bilateral bony defect (*arrows*) is present in this patient. Only a small posterior ossicle remains. (**c**) Note the defect of the posterior arch of C1 (*arrow*). The arch itself is underdeveloped, and the residual ossicles are tapered and triangular in configuration. (**d**) Total absence of the posterior arch of C1 (*arrows*). (**e**) Axial CT study shows absence of the posterior arch of C1 (*arrows*). All of these patients had stable cervical spines

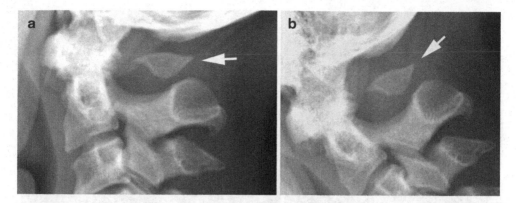

Fig. 3.16 C1 posterior arch defect: demonstration of stability. (**a**) Note the underdeveloped posterior arch of C1 with only a small triangular piece of bone remaining (*arrow*). Note its relationship to the neural arch of C2. (**b**) With flexion there is no change in the relationship of the residual bony ossicle (*arrow*) and the neural arch of C2. The spine is stable. Note the degenerative changes in the midcervical spine in this patient. This patient was a 75-year-old male. How many times do you think he flexed, extended, rotated, twisted his neck in 75 years and yet, it remained stable?

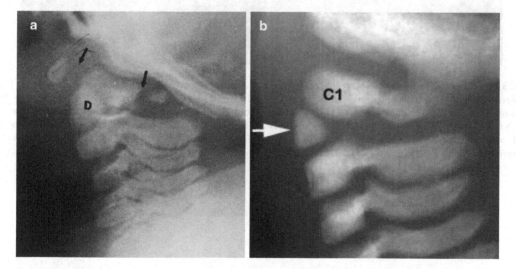

Fig. 3.17 Complex upper cervical spine anomalies. (**a**) Note the extensive defect/dysplasia of the posterior arch of C1 (*posterior arrow*). The predental distance (*anterior arrow*) is markedly increased. The dens (D) is hypoplastic. (**b**) In this patient the dens is hypoplastic (*arrow*). The lateral mass of C1 (C1) is overgrown and there is no anterior arch of C1. The neural arches of C2 and C3 show partial fusion

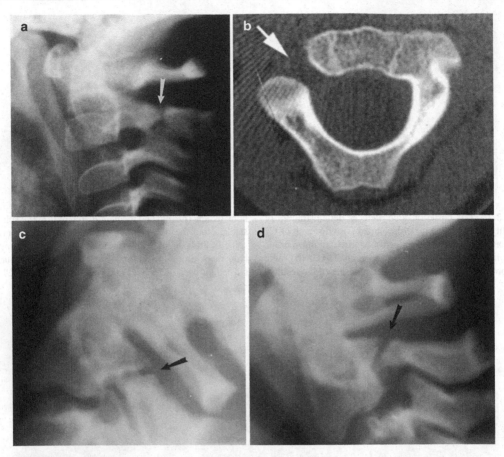

Fig. 3.18 C2 posterior arch defects. (**a**) Note that the posterior arch of C2 is unusually long and slightly dysplastic. There is a congenital defect (*arrow*) present. (**b**) Axial CT in another patient demonstrates a unilateral congenital defect (*arrow*) with smooth sclerotic margins. (**c**) Another patient. Note the defect (*arrow*) of the posterior arch of C2. Sclerosis is present on both sides. (**d**) On flexion there is no change in the configuration or width of the defect (*arrow*) ((**c**, **d**) From LE Swischuk, *Emergency Imaging of the Acutely Ill or Injured Child*, 4th ed. Lippincott Williams & Wilkins, Baltimore, 2000)

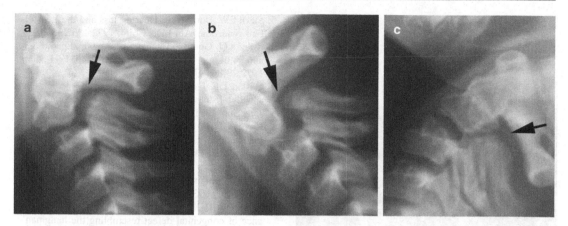

Fig. 3.19 Congenital defect of C2 associated with C2 dyplasia. (**a**) Note the defect (*arrow*) of the posterior arch of C2. The posterior arches of C2 and C3 are fused and dysplastic. In addition, there is some anterior displacement of the body of C2 and some widening of the anterior disk space. (**b**) With flexion the defect does not change (*arrow*). There is slight movement of C2 with reduction of the anterior disk width. (**c**) With extension the defect (*arrow*) closes slightly and the body of C2 lines up with the body of C3. The degree of motion was no more than 2 mm in this patient. Basically the spine is stable under ordinary activities. Caution might be used beyond ordinary activities

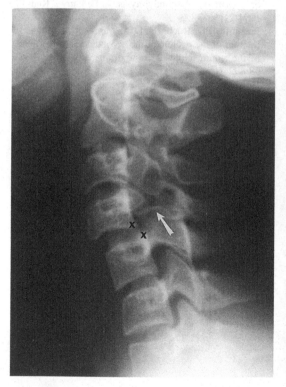

Fig. 3.20 Posterior neural arch defect, lower cervical spine. Note the congenital defect, with sclerotic edges (*arrow*) at the C4 level. As a result, C4 is anteriorly displaced on C5 (*cross symbols*)

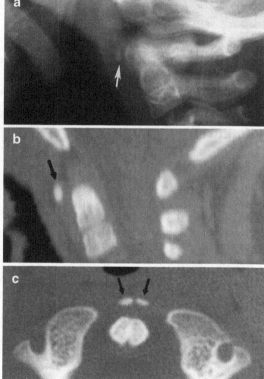

Fig. 3.21 Hypoplastic anterior arch C1. (**a**) Note that the anterior arch is very small (*arrow*). (**b**) Sagittal reconstructed CT demonstrates the hypoplastic anterior arch (*arrow*). (**c**) Axial CT study demonstrates two hypoplastic ossicles (*arrows*)

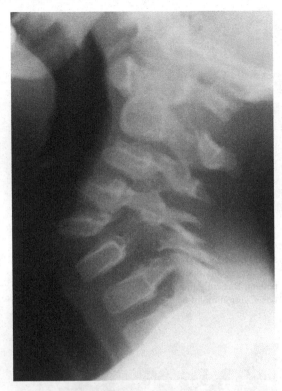

Fig. 3.22 Neural arch dysplasia. In this patient, extensive dysplasia of the neural arches results in angular lordosis of the midcervical spine. There is associated vertebral body underdevelopment

References

1. Nisan N, Hiz M, Saner H. Total agenesis of five cervical vertebrae: brief report. J Bone Joint Surg Br. 1988;70:668–9.
2. Fielden P, Russell JGB. Coronally cleft vertebra. Clin Radiol. 1970;21:327–8.
3. Palant DI, Carter BL. Klippel–Feil syndrome and deafness. A study with polytomography. Am J Dis Child. 1972;123:218–21.
4. Ramsey J, Bliznak J. Klippel–Feil syndrome with renal agenesis and other anomalies. Am J Roentgenol. 1971;113:460–3.
5. Stark EW, Borton TE. Hearing loss and the Klippel–Feil syndrome. Am J Dis Child. 1972;123:233–5.
6. Robain O, Gorce F. Iniencephaly: clinical pathologic and etiologic study of 13 cases. Arch Fr Pediatr. 1972;29:861–79.
7. Fardon DF, Fielding JW. Defects of the pedicle and spondylolisthesis of the second cervical vertebra. J Bone Joint Surg Br. 1981;63:526–8.
8. Riebel GD, Bayley JC. A congenital defect resembling the hangman's fracture. Spine. 1991;16:1240–1.
9. Smith JRT, Skoinner SR, Shonnard NH. Persistent synchondrosis of the second cervical vertebra simulating a hangman's fracture in a child. J Bone Joint Surg Am. 1993;75A:1228–30.
10. Williams III JP, Baker DH, Miller WA. CT appearance of congenital defect resembling the hangman's fracture. Pediatr Radiol. 1999;29:549–50.
11. Nordstrom REA, Lahdenranta TV, Kaitila II, Laasonen EMI. Familial spondylolisthesis of the axis vertebra. J Bone Joint Surg Br. 1986;68:704–6.
12. Currarino G. Primary spondylolysis of the axis vertebra (C2) in three children, including one with pylenocysostosis. Pediatr Radiol. 1989;19:535–8.
13. Parisi M, Lieberson R, Statsky S. Hangman's fracture or primary spondylolysis. Pediatr Radiol. 1991;21:367–8.
14. Pizzutillo PD, Rocha E, D'Astous J, et al. Bilateral fracture of the pedicle of the second cervical vertebra in the young child. J Bone Joint Surg Am. 1986;68:892–6.
15. Howard AW, Letts RM. Cervical spondylolysis in children: is it posttraumatic? J Pediatr Orthop. 2000;20:677–81.
16. Keinman PK. Hangman's fracture in an abused infant: imaging features. Pediatr Radiol. 1997;27:776–7.
17. Charlton OP, Gehweiller JA, Morgan CL, et al. Spondylolysis and spondylolisthesis of the cervical spine. Skeletal Radiol. 1978;3:79–84.
18. Forsberg DA, Martinez S, Vogler J, et al. Cervical spondylolysis: imaging findings in twelve patients. AJR Am J Roentgenol. 1990;154:751–5.
19. Prioleau GR, Wilson C. Cervical spondylolysis with spondylolisthesis. J Neurosurg. 1975;43:750–3.
20. Archer E, Batniotzky S, Franken EA, et al. Congenital dysplasia of C2–C6. Pediatr Radiol. 1977;6:121–2.
21. Saltzman CL, Hensinger RN, Blane CE, Phillips WA. Familial cervical dysplasia. J Bone Joint Surg Am. 1991;73:163–71.

Anomalies and Normal Variations of the Dens

4

The Os Terminale–Os Odontoideum Complex

There always has been some disagreement about whether the os terminale and the os odontoideum are the same or different bones. However, *I have always considered them to be the same, believing that the os terminale becomes the os odontoideum when it enlarges in association with hypoplasia of the dens* [1]. This also has been suggested by others [2], and the concept is depicted in Fig. 4.1.

Embryologically, the os terminale is derived from the fourth occipital sclerotome and eventually fuses with the dens, as shown earlier in Fig. 4.1. If, on the other hand, the dens undergoes hypoplasia, the os terminale overgrows and becomes the os odontoideum (Fig. 4.1). What is important about all this is that the os odontoideum, as it enlarges, can assume an almost endless, and often very bizarre, variety of configurations. At the same time, there is underdevelopment of the ligaments stabilizing C1 and C2, and because of this the whole problem is associated with varying degrees of hypermobility and instability of C1 and C2, frequently requiring surgical stabilization.

The normal os terminale sits atop the dens in a V-shaped notch (Fig. 4.2), and in some cases its location is more posterior than anterior (Fig. 4.3). In some of these cases the os terminale is a little larger than usual. When the os terminale is seated deep within the notch of the dens, it is not seen on lateral view, but in other cases it sits well above the tip of the dens and appears as a single, smooth ossicle (Fig. 4.4a). In some of these cases the dens is a little dysplastic/deformed in appearance but not overtly hypoplastic (Fig. 4.4b). In other cases, especially on CT evaluation, confusing, but still normal, bony fragmentation of the dens may mimic a comminuted dens fracture (Fig. 4.5). In this regard, however, one might recall that extensively comminuted fractures of the tip of the dens are basically nonexistent.

As noted earlier, when the dens becomes hypoplastic, the os terminale enlarges and overgrows to become the os odontoideum. The os odontoideum can be relatively small or very large, round or oval, or very bizarre and irregular in appearance. At any rate, when this complex of findings is seen the upper cervical spine becomes unstable (Figs. 4.6 and 4.7). Generally, if there is forward flexion motion of C1 on C2 greater than 2 mm, pathologic instability is present. Surgical stabilization is required, and this is important because *many, of these cases are incidentally discovered in the Emergency Room when trauma to the head and/or cervical spine has been sustained.* Therefore, while in some cases the findings may be minor and of no clinical consequence, in other instances significant instability of the upper cervical spine is present and the problem becomes just as great as if an unstable fracture were present.

In addition, the os odontoideum can be found posterior to its normal location, just as the normal

L.E. Swischuk, *Imaging of the Cervical Spine in Children*,
DOI 10.1007/978-1-4614-3788-8_4, © Springer Science+Business Media New York 2013

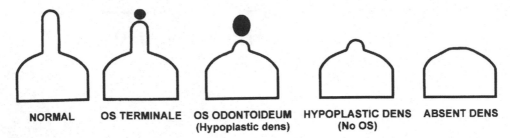

NORMAL   OS TERMINALE   OS ODONTOIDEUM   HYPOPLASTIC DENS   ABSENT DENS
                                (Hypoplastic dens)   (No OS)

Fig. 4.1 Range of dens anomalies. *Left* to *right*: normal dens with a fused os terminale; normal dens with an unfused os terminale; hypoplastic dens with an enlarged unfused os terminale (now termed an os odontoideum); hypoplasia of the dens with no development of the os terminale; complete absence of the dens (Modified from von Torklus D, Gehle W. The Upper Cervical Spine: Regional Morphology, Pathology, and Traumatology; An X-Ray Atlas. New York: Grune & Stratton; 1972)

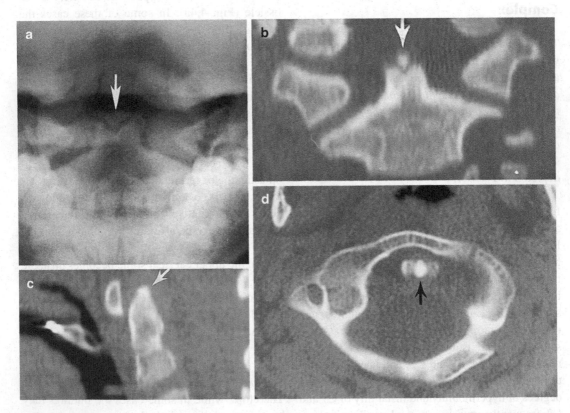

Fig. 4.2 Normal os terminale. (**a**) Note the os terminale (*arrow*) embedded into the V-shaped notch of the dens. (**b**) Similar findings; os terminale (*arrow*) on a coronally reconstructed CT study. (**c**) Sagittal CT reconstruction demonstrates the typical position of the os terminale (*arrow*). (**d**) Axial CT study demonstrates the usual central position of the os terminale (*arrow*)

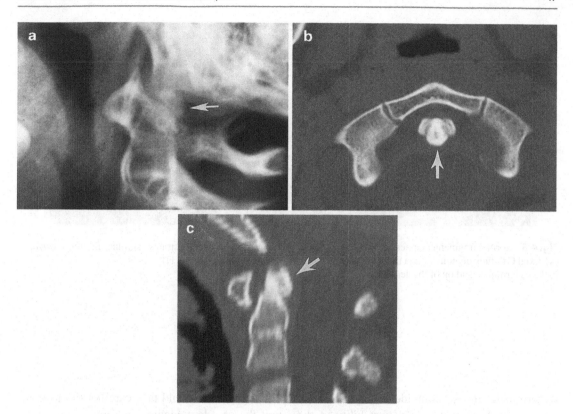

Fig. 4.3 Normal os terminale: posterior position. (**a**) Slightly large, posteriorly located os terminale (*arrow*). (**b**) Axial CT study in another patient demonstrates the os terminale (*arrow*) to be slightly posterior in location. (**c**) Sagittal reconstruction view more clearly demonstrates the posterior location of the os terminale (*arrow*)

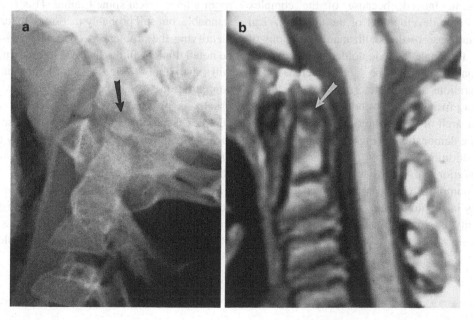

Fig. 4.4 Normal os terminale. (**a**) Note the normal os terminale (*arrow*), high sitting atop the normally developed dens. (**b**) Sagittal tomogram in another patient demonstrates the round os terminale (*arrow*) sitting atop the short dens

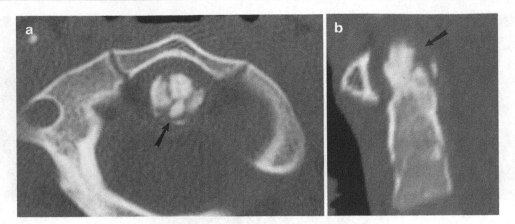

Fig. 4.5 Normal fragmented appearance of os terminale. (**a**) Axial CT study demonstrates a fragmented appearance to the os terminale and tip of the dens (*arrow*). (**b**) Sagittal reconstruction demonstrates similar findings (*arrow*) (From Swischuk et al. [1])

os terminale. In os odontoideum cases one can presume that some degree of instability of the upper cervical spine may be present (Fig. 4.8). In addition, the anterior arch of C1 can overgrow and falsely suggest that an ununited dens fracture is present. Indeed, because of the complex embryologic development of the upper cervical spine and base of the skull, many variations of the os terminale–os odontoideum complex of abnormalities can be encountered. The configurations of these abnormalities are endless, including fusing of the os odontoideum with the anterior arch of C1 or the occiput, and some of these are demonstrated (Figs. 4.9 and 4.10).

In addition to the foregoing abnormal configurations of the os terminale–os odontoideum complex, one can encounter abnormal ossicles in the area (Fig. 4.11). Furthermore, if instability is significant, cord compression can result (Fig. 4.12).

Finally, one should take care not to misinterpret the os odontoideum for a missed odontoid fracture [3] for the findings are different (see Fig. 4.14). Such an error can occur because very often these cases are first identified in the emergency room after cervical spine trauma. This is understandable, but still probably incorrect. In terms of identifying the problem as congenital, it should be noted that (1) all the involved bony structures will have smooth edges, and (2) the anatomic configuration of the bony structures involved usually is bizarre. Of course, since the whole complex is variably unstable, superimposed cervical spine trauma can render a previously quasi-unstable configuration more unstable and, in fact, able to lead to acute cord injury.

Finally, a word is in order regarding the acquired os odontoideum [4, 5], where initial trauma interrupts the blood supply to the dens. Most often such trauma consists of a flexion-

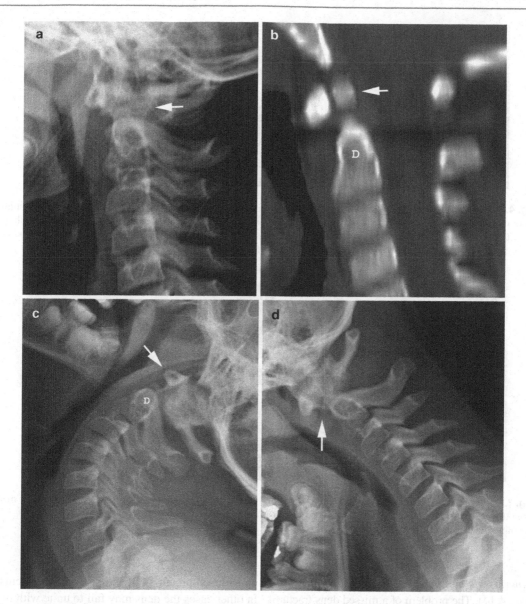

Fig. 4.6 Hypoplastic dens, os odontoideum, and hypermobility. (**a**) The dens is not clearly visualized (*arrow*). The reason is that it is hypoplastic. (**b**) Sagittal reconstructed CT image demonstrates the hypoplastic dens (D) and the os odontoideum (*arrow*). Note the relationship of the anterior arch of C1 to the dens. (**c**) With extension the anterior arch of C1 (*arrow*) comes to lie directly over the dens (D). (**d**) With flexion the anterior arch of C1 moves far forward and the space between it and the dens becomes markedly widened (*arrow*)

induced injury with anterior displacement of C1 on C2 and fracturing and anterior displacement of the dens. In time, the dens resorbs, and the normal os terminale overgrows to become an acquired os odontoideum (Fig. 4.13).

Neither the congenital nor the acquired os odontoideum should be confused with an ununited dens fracture. In the latter case the dens is normal in size and configuration, but since there is nonunion through the base of the dens, it becomes

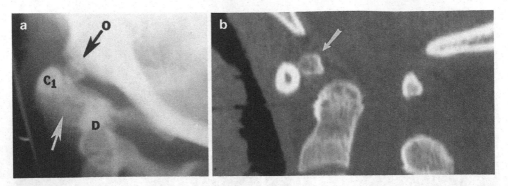

Fig. 4.7 Hypoplastic dens, os odontoideum, and hypermobility. (**a**) Note the markedly widened C1-dens distance (*white arrow*). The dens (D) is hypoplastic. C1 (C₁) is slightly enlarged and the os odontoideum (O) is anteriorly dislocated. (**b**) Sagittal reconstructed CT study in another patient demonstrates findings similar to those seen in (**a**). Note the small, anteriorly displaced os odontoideum (*arrow*)

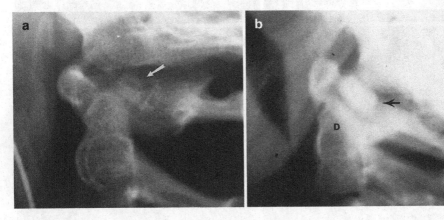

Fig. 4.8 Posterior positioning of the os odontoideum. (**a**) Note the posterior position of the round os odontoideum (*arrow*). The dens is a little hypoplastic. (**b**) In this patient the posteriorly positioned large os odontoideum is oval (*arrow*). The dens (D) is hypoplastic

hypermobile and behaves like an os odontoideum (Fig. 4.14). The problem of a missed dens fracture is not as common as it was in the past because today more initial attention is paid to the cervical spine in acute trauma. In the end, however, whether the dens is hypermobile because of an old, ununited fracture, or congenitally, unstable, the findings mitigate toward the need for surgical stabilization.

Absence of the Dens

The dens can fail to develop entirely [6], resulting in hypermobility of the upper cervical spine (Fig. 4.15). The dens simply is missing in these patients; but of more importance is the marked underdevelopment of the associated ligaments. In other cases the dens may fail to unite with the body of C2 and remain as the body of C1 (Fig. 4.16). At first these cases may be confusing, but once one understands the embryologic development of the upper cervical spine and base of the occiput, one can methodically analyze the findings and determine the true congenital origin of the anomaly.

Tilting of the Dens

Normal tilting of the dens can cause problems in terms of differentiation from findings that occur with true fractures of the dens. In this regard, the

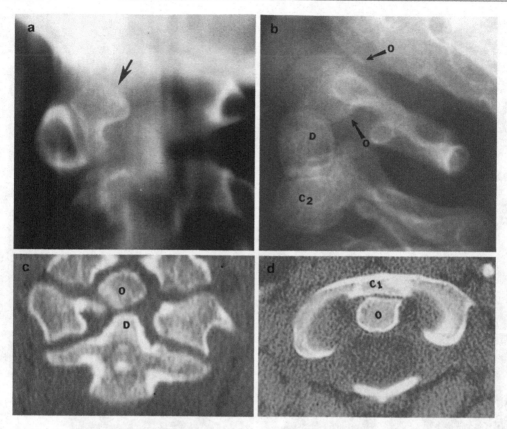

Fig. 4.9 Os odontoideum: various configurations. (**a**) Tomogram demonstrating a peculiarly shaped os odontoideum (*arrow*), articulating with an enlarged anterior arch of C1. (**b**) In this patient, the large, round os odontoideum (O) is sitting above the hypoplastic dens (D). Body of C2 (C$_2$). (**c**) Another patient with a large os odontoideum (O) sitting on a hypoplastic dens (D). (**d**) Same patient demonstrating the large os odontoideum (O) articulating with the anterior arch of C1 (C$_1$)

dens, on a normal basis, is frequently posteriorly tilted [7]. If one is not aware of this configuration, however, it could be misinterpreted as a fracture (Fig. 4.17).

Anterior tilting of the dens, on a normal basis, is far less common (Fig. 4.18a). Most often anterior tilting of the dens is the result of a fracture through the dens-body synchondrosis of C2. Normal lateral tilting also can occur. This configuration is now very common with the patient on the backboard during an EMS delivery. Therefore, as opposed to the past, the dens now frequently appears laterally tilted on CT and plain film imaging studies (Fig. 4.18b, c).

Bifed Dens

The dens forms from two lateral masses and the os terminale at its tip. If the two lateral masses fail to unite, a bifed dens results [8]. This anomaly usually is best seen on coronally reconstructed CT studies of the upper cervical spine (Fig. 4.19), and is stable.

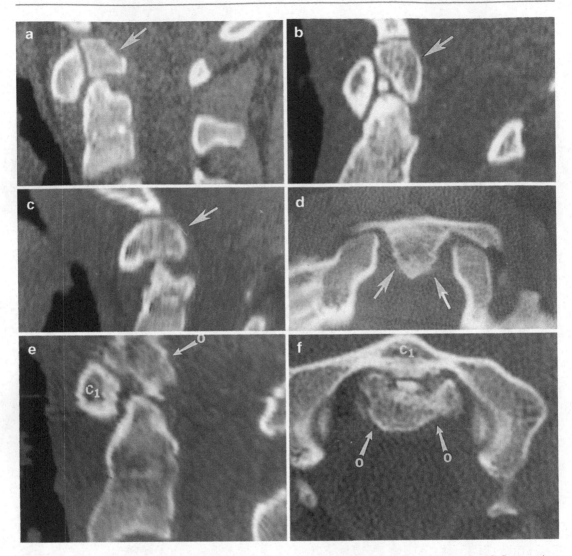

Fig. 4.10 Os odontoideum: various configurations. (**a**) Note the irregular os odontoideum (*arrow*), articulating with the anterior arch of C1. The dens is hypoplastic. (**b**) In this patient the large irregular os odontoideum (*arrow*) is nearly fused with the occiput above it. A small ossicle is present between the os odontoideum and the anterior arch of C1. The dens is hypoplastic. (**c**) The os odontoideum (*arrow*) in this patient is fused with the anterior arch of

C1. The dens is hypoplastic and irregular. (**d**) Same patient demonstrating the os odontoideum (*arrows*) fused with the anterior arch of C1. (**e**) The os odontoideum (O) is very large and irregular. Anterior arch of C1 (C_1). The dens is hypoplastic. (**f**) Axial view demonstrates the large, irregular os odontoideum (O) articulating, and indeed almost fused with, the anterior arch of C1 (C_1)

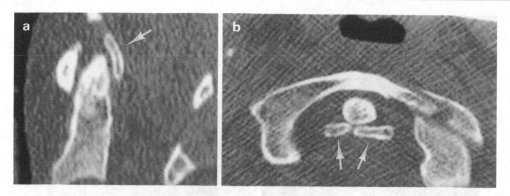

Fig. 4.11 Hypoplastic dens; bizarre accessory ossicles. (a) Note the bizarre, oval-shaped ossicle (*arrow*) posterior to the slightly hypoplastic dens. (b) Axial view demonstrates two ossicles (*arrows*), located posterior to the hypoplastic dens

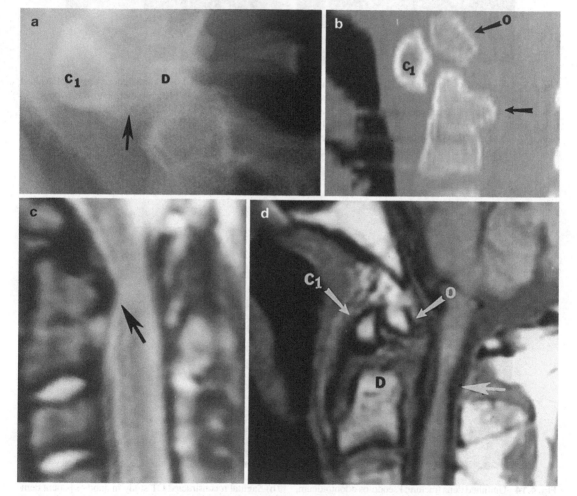

Fig. 4.12 Os odontoideum complex with spinal cord involvement. (a) In this patient note the wide predental distance (*arrow*), hypertrophied anterior arch of C1 (C_1), and the hypoplastic dens (D). The os odontoideum is barely visible. (b) Sagittal reconstructed CT study demonstrates the large os odontoideum (Os). The anterior arch of C1 is hypertrophied (C_1) while the dens is underdeveloped. A peculiar osteophyte is present along the posterior aspect of the dens (*arrow*). (c) MR study, T2 weighted. Note compression of the spinal cord (*arrow*). (d) In this patient there is marked cord atrophy (*arrow*) resulting from chronic injury to the spinal cord. Anterior arch of C1 (C_1), os odontoideum (O), and hypoplastic dens (D)

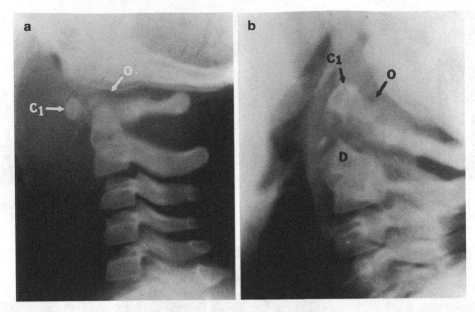

Fig. 4.13 Acquired os odontoideum. (**a**) Note the anteriorly (dislocated) anterior arch of C1 (C$_1$). The predental distance is increased, and there is considerable prevertebral soft tissue swelling. The os terminale (O) is slightly anteriorly displaced (dislocated). (**b**) Months later there has been resorption of the dens (D), and the os terminale (O) has overgrown to become an acquired os odontoideum. A residual avulsed bony fragment also is present anterior to the hypoplastic dens (D). Anterior arch of C1 (C$_1$) (Reprinted with permission Ricciardi JE, Kaufer H, Louis DS. Acquired os odontoideum following acute ligament injury: Report of a case. J Bone Joint Surg Am 1976;58a:410–412)

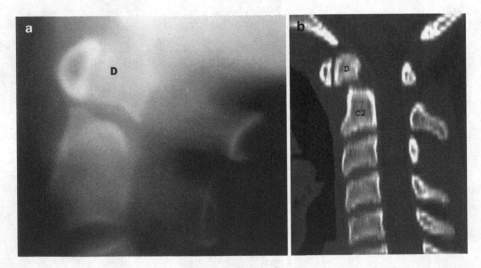

Fig. 4.14 Ununited dens fracture; Pseudo-os odontoideum. (**a**) Note the ununited dens fracture. The dens is normal in size and bulk. However, it is not fused to the underlying body of C2 and was the result of an ununited dens fracture. (**b**) Sagittal reconstructed CT study in another patient demonstrates the mobile dens (D) which is normal in size and configuration. However, it is not fused to the underlying body of C2 and was the result of an ununited dens fracture

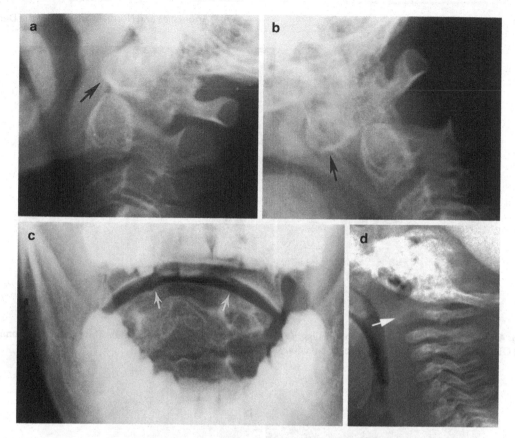

Fig. 4.15 Absent dens. (**a**) Note the large bony structure (*arrow*), which at first might be misinterpreted as an ununited dens. (**b**) With flexion, however, it can be seen that the bony structure actually is the overgrown anterior arch of C1 (*arrow*) and that there is no dens. Only the body of C2 is visualized. (**c**) The open-mouth odontoid demonstrates that the superior aspect of the body of C2 is smooth (*arrows*) and that there is no dens. (**d**) Newborn with absence of the dens (*arrow*)

Fig. 4.16 Dens as body of C1. The dens (D) is separated from the body of C2 and fused with the posterior arch of C1. It actually now becomes the body of C1. The ossicle above is the overgrown os terminale, now termed the os odontoideum (O)

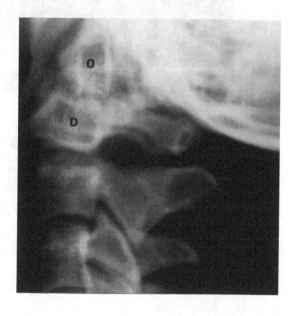

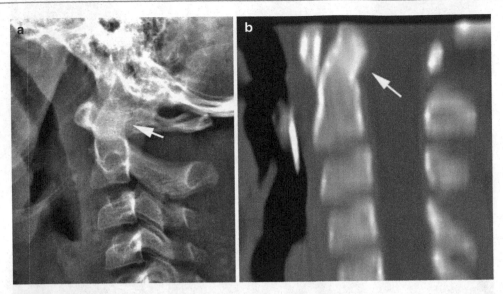

Fig. 4.17 Posteriorly tilted dens: normal finding. (**a**) Note the posteriorly tilted dens (D). This patient was normal. (**b**) CT study, sagittal reconstruction. Note the posteriorly tilted dens (*arrow*)

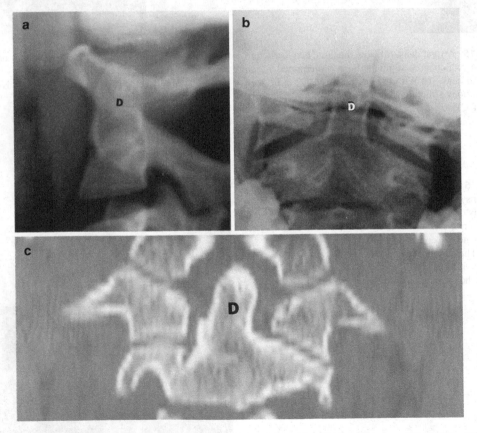

Fig. 4.18 Anterior and lateral tilting of the dens. (**a**) Note normal anterior tilting of the dens (D). (**b**) Normal lateral tilting of the dens (D). (**c**) Axial CT study lateral tilting of the dens (D)

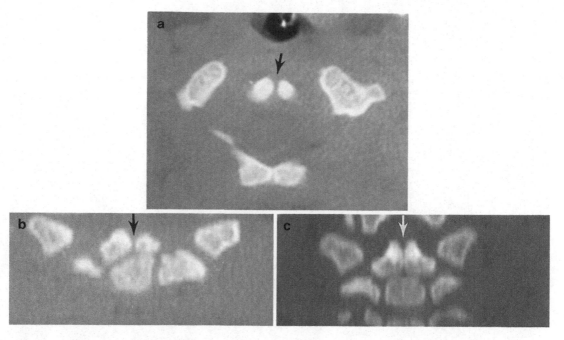

Fig. 4.19 Bifed dens. (**a**) Note the bifed dens (*arrow*). (**b**) Coronal reconstruction again demonstrates the bifed dens (*arrow*). (**c**) Another patient with a bifed dens (*arrow*)

References

1. Swischuk LE, John SD, Moorthy C. The os terminale–os odontoideum complex. Emerg Radiol. 1997;4:72–81.
2. von Torklus D, Gehle W. The upper cervical spine: regional morphology, pathology, and traumatology; an X-ray atlas. New York: Grune & Stratton; 1972.
3. Kuhns LR, Loder RT, Farley FA, Hensinger RN. Nuchal cord changes in children with os odontoideum: evidence for associated trauma. J Pediatr Orthop. 1998;18:815–9.
4. Hawkins RJ, Fielding JW, Thompson WJ. Os odontoideum: congenital or acquired: a case report. J Bone Joint Surg Am. 1976;58:413–4.
5. Ricciardi JE, Kaufer H, Louis DS. Acquired os odontoideum following acute ligament injury: report of a case. J Bone Joint Surg Am. 1976;58a:410–2.
6. Gwinn JL, Smith JL. Acquired and congenital absence of the odontoid process. Am J Roentgenol Radium Ther Nucl Med. 1962;88:424–31.
7. Swischuk LE, Hayden Jr CK, Sarwar M. The posteriorly tilted dens is normal variation mimicking a fracture of the dens. Pediatr Radiol. 1979;8:27–8.
8. Garant M, Oudjhane K, Sinsky A, O'Gorman AM. Duplicated odontoid process: plain radiographic and CT appearance of a rare congenital anomaly of the cervical spine. AJNR Am J Neuroradiol. 1997;18:1719–20.

Trauma

5

Introduction

Mechanisms of injury of the cervical spine are the same in infants and young children as in adults, but the results may be different. Older children and adolescents can be considered adults in terms of types and locations of fractures. Overall, more fractures are induced by flexion forces than by extension forces, and in this regard, because the apex of the flexion curve in infants and young children is through the upper cervical spine [1], it is not a surprise that more fractures occur at this level than lower in the cervical spine [2–5]. Thereafter, as the child grows older, and into adolescence, the apex of the flexion curve is transferred to the midcervical spine as shown earlier (see Fig. 2.4). As a result, injuries become more common at this level.

Forces Involved in Cervical Spine Injury

Basically there are four forces involved in trauma to the cervical spine: flexion, extension, rotational, and axial loading forces (Fig. 5.1). Flexion and anterior rotational injuries are more common than extension and posterior rotational injuries. Pure axial loading injuries are less common than any of the foregoing types of injuries, *but in any given case, more than one force often is at play.* Nonetheless, it is important to appreciate that each of these forces leads to definitive patterns of injury, both bony and soft tissue. In fact, detailed *analysis of the initial lateral cervical spine radiograph usually allows one to deduce, from the abnormalities detected, which forces were involved.*

Plain Film Views Required

Before the advent of computerized tomography, a complete five-view cervical spine series usually was obtained. This consisted of AP, lateral, both oblique, and open-mouth odontoid views of the cervical spine, but in actual fact, the two views that were most productive were the lateral and open-mouth odontoid views. The swimmer's view was frequently added to visualize the lower cervical spine, but currently, if there is difficulty visualizing this portion of the cervical spine, CT evaluation is obtained. As a result, on initial investigation of cervical spine trauma the lateral cervical spine and open-mouth odontoid views are most important. However, in infants and young children, obtaining proper plain films can be a problem, especially the open-mouth odontoid view [6]. Generally speaking, if the upper cervical spine or the lower cervical spine is not adequately visualized on the lateral and open-mouth odontoid views, one probably should proceed to CT examination of these areas. This generally leads to rapid disposition of the problem, *but in infants and children aged 5 years and under, such CT studies may not be required.* This is especially

L.E. Swischuk, *Imaging of the Cervical Spine in Children*,
DOI 10.1007/978-1-4614-3788-8_5, © Springer Science+Business Media New York 2013

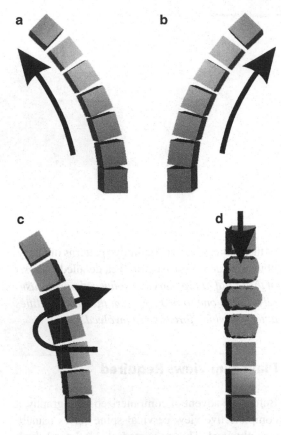

Fig. 5.1 Forces encountered in trauma to the spine. (**a**) Flexion forces. (**b**) Extension forces. (**c**) Rotational forces. (**d**) Axial compression forces

true of the upper cervical spine, where a normal lateral cervical spine view may suffice [6].

In our institution we attempt to obtain a proper open-mouth odontoid view twice, but if the second attempt fails, and clinical/radiographic suspicion of injury is low and the lateral view normal, we stop the study. This is possible because in infants and young children, odontoid fractures generally occur through the synchondrosis between the dens and the body of C2 [7–9], and thus, almost invariably the presence of such a fracture can be excluded on lateral views of the cervical spine. Clearly, if this cannot be accomplished, one should proceed to CT evaluation, but most often one can feel secure with a normal lateral and open-mouth odontoid view [6]. This is

not true of the lower cervical spine, for if the lower cervical spine is not visualized and the presence of injury in this area is suspected, one should proceed to CT imaging.

Additional Imaging of Cervical Spine Trauma

There is no question that most initial information regarding serious cervical spine injuries can be obtained from the lateral cervical spine and open-mouth odontoid views, if one knows how to evaluate them. However, CT imaging, with reconstruction in various planes, is mandatory for further evaluation and also is useful in detecting otherwise occult fractures of the cervical spine and base of the skull [10–14]. It should be noted, however, that many of these latter fractures are not important in terms of cervical spine instability. Indeed, when these injuries are identified it is important to convey their proper significance to the referring physician, and their family. The reason for this is that to the lay public, any mention of a cervical spine fracture results in considerable anxiety. *It is important, therefore, to indicate to people who consult us that while certain injuries are critical and unstable and need immediate attention, others, although still important and painful, are not unstable, will not result in a serious consequence, and will resolve with time.*

Magnetic resonance imaging also is useful in acute trauma, but it generally is used in selected cases. Basically, it should be used when cord injury is suspected on the basis of clinical or imaging findings. There is no question that MRI is excellent in delineating spinal cord and soft tissue injury, but it should be used only when information regarding these anatomic regions is required.

Finally, in any case plain films can be augmented by obtaining flexion–extension views [15]. However, in one study [16], it was determined that if the lateral and open-mouth odontoid views were normal, flexion–extension views offered very little further information. This point notwithstanding, there still are instances in which the flexion view will demonstrate a formerly occult posterior ligament injury. Of course, flexion views should not be obtained when initial plain film examination clearly shows instability of the spine.

Flexion views can be obtained in cooperative patients with the patient flexing his or her neck on request. In less cooperative patients, and indeed in unconscious patients, flexion views of the cervical spine still can be obtained *if the radiologist flexes the spine in increments.* Each flexion maneuver should be recorded with a portable film, and once this has been analyzed and it has been determined that no abnormality is present, the neck can be flexed slightly more. Eventually, full flexion will be obtained, and one can determine whether an underlying injury is present.

Plain Film Signs of Cervical Spine Instability

Signs of cervical spine instability may be very graphic and florid or extremely subtle. It is important that one becomes thoroughly familiar with all these signs, both on plain films and on CT. These are dealt with in more detail throughout this chapter, but an overall view is presented in Table 5.1. In this regard, *the most important job for the initial observer of the cervical spine imaging study is to determine whether cervical spine instability is present* [17, 18]. *There is no question that although many minor injuries result in prolonged pain and discomfort to the patient, and the patient may not consider the pain to be minor, the most important task to be accomplished when first inspecting the cervical spine plain film series is to determine whether cervical spine instability is present.*

Specific Injuries

It is important to understand the underlying mechanics of the various injuries sustained in the cervical spine, and to this end, cervical spine

Table 5.1 Signs of cervical spine instability

Finding	Mechanism of injury
Anterior vertebral body displacement	Flexion, anterior rotation
Posterior vertebral body displacement	Extension, posterior rotation
Disk space narrowing	Flexion, anterior rotation
Disk space widening	Extension, posterior rotation
Teardrop fracture	Flexion, extension
V-shaped apophyseal joints	Flexion, anterior rotation
Wide apophyseal joints	Flexion, rotation
Dislocated apophyseal joints	Flexion, anterior rotation
Offset or locked apophyseal joints	Flexion, anterior rotation
Bilateral pars fracture	Extension
Increased interspinous distance	Flexion
Increased predental distance	Flexion, anterior rotation
Offset lateral masses of C1	Axial loading
Burst (fat) vertebra	Axial loading
Dens fractures	Flexion, extension, rotation
Prevertebral swelling	Flexion, extension, rotation

injuries are discussed, by mechanism, under the following headings: lower cervical spine (C3–C7) injuries and upper cervical spine (C1 and C2) injuries. The mechanisms of flexion, extension, lateral flexion, rotational, and axial compression have been illustrated earlier (Fig. 5.1), and it might be noted that in many cases more than one mechanism is at play.

Lower Cervical Spine Injuries

Flexion Force Induced Injuries

In older children, injuries of the lower cervical spine induced by flexion most commonly occur in the midportion of the spine. Characteristically with flexion forces there is anterior compression and posterior distraction. The compressive forces are dissipated through the vertebral body (usually

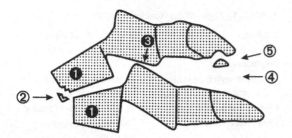

Fig. 5.2 Flexion force induced injuries: diagrammatic representation. With flexion, anterior compression forces result in wedge-like compression of the vertebral body (1), teardrop fractures (2), disruption of the apophyseal joints (3), and widening of the intraspinous distance (4), with or without avulsion fractures (5). Also note that the superior vertebral body is anteriorly displaced on the inferior vertebral body

the anterior portion), and distraction forces are dissipated through the apophyseal joints and ligaments between the spinous processes and neural arches (Fig. 5.2). Anterior vertebral body compression can be seen with or without an associated avulsion, inferior corner, teardrop fracture. This fracture results when the anterior longitudinal ligament is stretched and pulls off a piece of bone [19]. In children, this fragment often comes from the ring epiphysis [20]. Distracting forces posteriorly cause the neural arches to separate so that the intraspinous distance increases [21], with or without associated avulsion fractures (Fig. 5.2). In addition, similar ligament disruption can cause the posterior aspect of the disk space to widen as well. Overall, however, the intervening disk space usually is narrowed with flexion force induced injury (Figs. 5.3 and 5.4).

Anterior compression of the vertebral body also results in loss of vertebral body height and an anterior, wedge-like configuration, often involving the superior vertebral bony plate more than the inferior plate. Prevertebral soft tissue swelling is variable, and a teardrop fracture, usually involving the inferior, anterior corner of the vertebral body, often is present (Figs. 5.3 and 5.4). Increase in interspinous distance also can be seen on frontal views of the cervical spine [21], but it is so evident on lateral view that the frontal view findings are supplementary.

In more severe compressive injuries of the vertebral body, usually associated with some degree of axial loading, the vertebral body is crushed and expands in all directions (Fig. 5.5). The most important of these directions is posterior, for the bony fragments then encroach upon the spinal canal and compress the spinal cord. This phenomenon, to one degree or another, is common with flexion-induced compression fractures (Fig. 5.5). All the features of flexion-induced fractures of the vertebra, but especially the bony injuries are most vividly demonstrated with reconstructed CT studies, but for soft tissues and the spinal cord, MR imaging is best (Fig. 5.6).

Compression fractures of C3 are rare in any age group. However, they do occur, and the findings are no different from those associated with compression fractures occurring elsewhere (Fig. 5.7). In these cases, however, it is important to appreciate that although C3 may appear to be severely wedged, the wedging probably was present prior to the injury in the form of normal wedging.

Abnormalities of the apophyseal joints with flexion-induced injuries center around joint space disruption, and in some cases fracturing of the facettes and pedicles. These fractures are not readily detected on plain films and usually come to discovery on subsequent CT studies. On plain films the apophyseal joint can be separated and widened, or more importantly, V-shaped (Fig. 5.8). The superior facette also can slide forward on the inferior facette with less coverage of the inferior facette than normal (Fig. 5.8). In more severe cases the posterior corner of the superior facette becomes perched on the anterior corner of the inferior facette, leading to the "perched facette" sign (Fig. 5.9). With further anterior motion the superior facette jumps over the inferior facette and becomes locked on the inferior facette, constituting the "jumped" or "locked" facette sign (Fig. 5.10).

In some cases of flexion-induced injury no bony abnormality is evident, yet there is occult para-apophyseal joint and posterior interspinous ligament damage. This can be subtly apparent on initial lateral views of the cervical spine, as the interspinous distance will be slightly increased

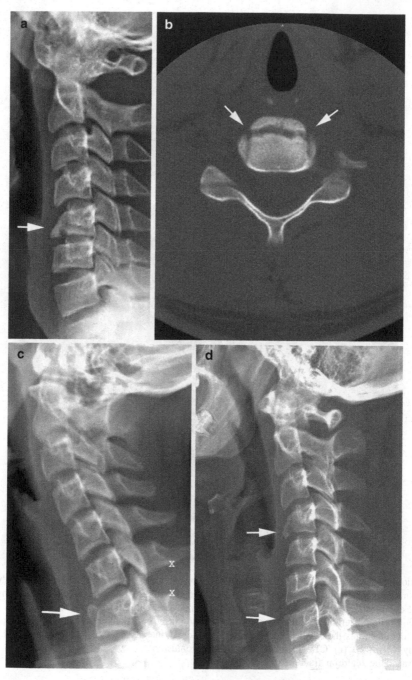

Fig. 5.3 Flexion-induced injuries: vertebral compression and teardrop fractures. (**a**) Note compression of C5 and a large teardrop fracture (*arrow*). There is no prevertebral soft tissue swelling. There may be very minimal widening of the apophyseal joint between C5 and C6. C5 is slightly retropulsed. (**b**) Axial CT demonstrates the compressed/fragmented vertebral body of C5 (*arrows*). (**c**) Another patient with anterior compression of C7, a teardrop fracture from the superior corner of the vertebral body (*arrow*), and widening of the intraspinous distance between C6 and C7 (X). The apophyseal joints are minimally widened and the superior facette slightly anteriorly positioned. (**d**) Another patient. Note teardrop fractures at two levels (*arrows*). At the upper level the teardrop arises from the inferior corner of the vertebral body. The vertebral body is compressed, minimally retropulsed and the disk space between it and the next vertebra (C5) is slightly narrowed. At the lower level, at C7, a superior corner teardrop fracture is noted and there is minimal compression of the vertebral body. The posterior elements and apophyseal joints appear normal. Again note that there is no prevertebral soft tissue swelling

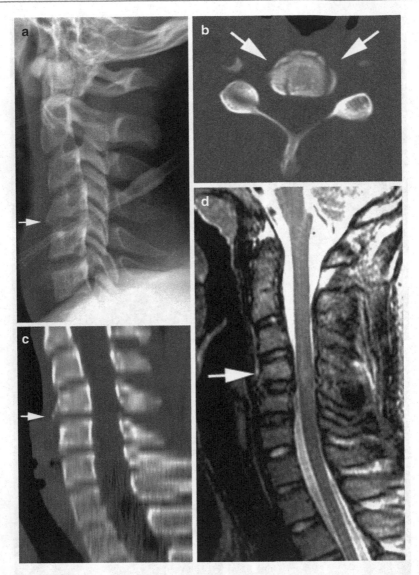

Fig. 5.4 Flexion-induced injuries: value of CT and MR. (a) Note the small anterior teardrop fracture (*arrow*) and the associated compressed vertebra (C4). There is minimal retropulsion. The posterior elements appear normal. (b) Axial CT demonstrates the crushed and fragmented vertebral body (*arrows*). (c) CT, Sagittal reconstruction demonstrates the teardrop fracture (*arrow*), slight compression of the vertebral body and slight retropulsion. (d) Sagittal MR T2 weighted study demonstrates slightly increased signal in the involved vertebral body (*arrow*), slight retropulsion, and widening of the spinal cord with some increased signal consistent with spinal cord contusion

and the apophyseal joints slightly widened, or even slightly V-shaped. In other cases, however, only subsequent flexion views will detect the underlying ligamentous instability (Fig. 5.11), and finally, avulsion fractures of the spinous tips can occur, and in the lower cervical spine these constitute the classic clay shoveler's fracture (Fig. 5.12).

Extension Force Induced Injuries

In the lower cervical spine, injuries induced by extension force tend to occur more at the C6–C7 level than in the midspine as seen with flexion force injuries. With extension force injuries, compressive forces are present posteriorly while distracting forces occur anteriorly (Fig. 5.13).

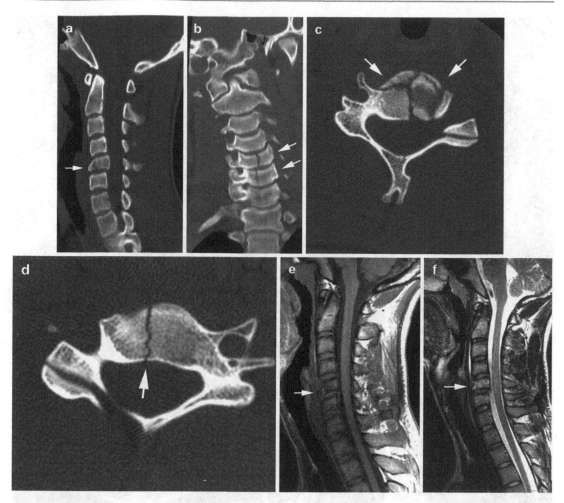

Fig. 5.5 Flexion-induced injuries: Value of CT and MR. (**a**) Sagittal reconstructed CT study demonstrates compression of C5, an anterior tear drop fracture, and a slight degree of retropulsion of C5 into the spinal canal (*arrow*). (**b**) Coronal reconstructed CT demonstrates that two vertebral bodies are involved (*arrows*). (**c**) Axial CT study of the upper vertebral body demonstrates complete crushing of the vertebral body (*arrows*). (**d**) Axial CT of the lower vertebral body demonstrates a single vertical fracture (*arrow*). (**e**) Sagittal MR, T1 weighted study demonstrates the compressed and slightly retropulsed vertebra and teardrop fracture (*arrow*). (**f**) Sagittal MR T2 weighted study demonstrates slightly increased signal in C5 (*arrow*). Also note the teardrop fracture. There is very minimal increase in signal in the vertebral body below (C6). There is slight retropulsion of C5. The cord appears a little thickened in the area and there is slightly increased signal consistent with a mild contusion

As a result, one can see anterior widening of the disk space [22] secondary to rupture of the anterior longitudinal ligaments (Fig. 5.13). At the same time a teardrop fracture can result from an avulsion of a corner of the vertebra by the anterior ligaments. Most often such fractures involve the upper anterior corner of the vertebra (Fig. 5.13). The apophyseal joints usually are not dislocated with this type of injury, but fracturing of the neural arch can occur. In addition, because of the posterior compressive forces present, leverage is applied to the neural arch and unilateral or bilateral pars fractures can occur.

In the classic hyperextension injury shown in Fig. 5.14, bilateral pars fractures are seen. In addition anterior widening of the concomitant

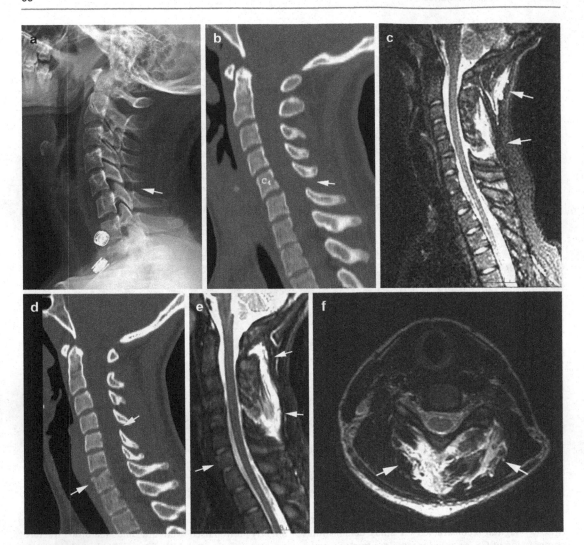

Fig. 5.6 Flexion-induced injuries, minimal plain film findings, value of CT and MR. (**a**) The cervical spine basically appears near normal. There is no soft tissue swelling. The only suspicious finding is slight increased in the interspinous distance between C5and C6 (*arrow*). The superior apophyseal joint facette also is slightly anteriorly positioned. (**b**) CT study sagittal reconstruction demonstrates the increased interspinous distance to be valid (*arrow*). In addition there is slight anterior displacement of C4 (C4) on C5. (**c**) Sagittal MR, T2 weighted study demonstrates extensive high signal in the upper posterior soft tissues consistent with a hyperflexion injury and dis-tracting forces posteriorly. (**d**) Another patient. Note compression of C6 along with a superior teardrop fracture (*arrow*). There may be slight soft tissue swelling causing bulging into the posterior wall of the trachea. At the level of C4 and C5 the interspinous distance appears increased (*posterior arrow*). (**e**) Sagittal MR T2 weighted study demonstrates slight increased signal in the body of C6 (*anterior arrow*) and extensive high signal of the soft tissues over the upper posterior cervical spine (*posterior arrow*). (**f**) MR axial T2 weighted study demonstrates the same posterior soft tissue edema along with low signal hematoma (*arrows*)

intervertebral disk space is as well as slight anterior subluxation of the upper vertebra. On CT imaging, pars fractures appear the same as they do in the upper cervical spine in the classic hangman's fracture (see later: Fig. 5.30).

Hyperextension injuries are notorious for producing injury (contusion) to the spinal cord without any visible bony or ligamentous injury. This has been termed the SCIWORA injury [23, 24] and in the past was known as the "central cord

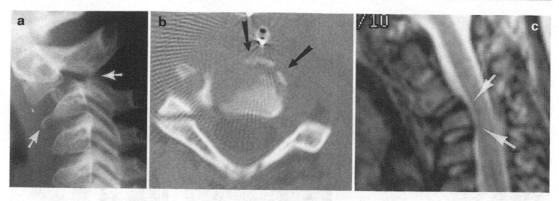

Fig. 5.7 Flexion force injury: less common location (C2–C3). (**a**) Note that C2 is anteriorly displaced on C3. There is an anterior avulsion (teardrop) fracture (*anterior arrow*). The prevertebral soft tissues are slightly prominent. The apophyseal joint between C2 and C3 is markedly disrupted, and the perched facette sign (*posterior arrow*) is present. (**b**) Axial CT study demonstrates the fragmented vertebral body of C3 (*arrows*). (**c**) Sagittal T2 MRI image demonstrates the posterior bulging of C3 into the spinal canal. The subarachnoid space is compromised, and there is slight indentation on the cord (*arrows*). No contusion is present. The wedge-shaped configuration of C3 in (**a**) probably is due not to the fracture but to a normal variation commonly seen in infants and young children (see Fig. 2.15) (Reproduced with permission from LE Swischuk, *Emergency Radiology of the Acutely Ill or Injured Child*, 4th ed. Lippincott Williams & Wilkins, Baltimore, 2000)

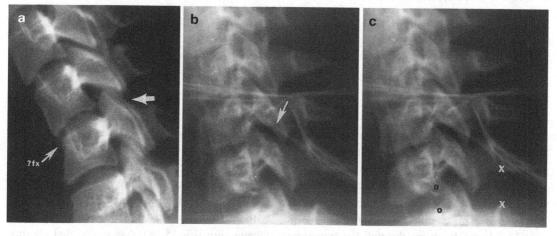

Fig. 5.8 Flexion-induced injury: apophyseal joint disruption. (**a**) Note the V-shaped apophyseal joint (*arrow*) and the anteriorly displaced superior facette. There is suggestion of minimal compression of the anterior superior aspect of the inferior vertebral body (?fx). (**b**) In this patient note the wide, slightly V-shaped apophyseal joint (*arrow*) and compare with the normal apophyseal joint above it. The apophyseal joint below it also is disrupted and the joint space widened. (**c**) Additional findings include posterior widening of the intervertebral disk space (Os) and widening of the intrasponous distance (X)

syndrome." In these cases, definite neurologic deficit referable to the lower cervical cord is present, and yet there is virtually nothing to see on plain films. In these cases, with hyperextension, buckling of the intracanalicular spinal ligaments results in cord compression and contusion. Magnetic resonance imaging is necessary for demonstrating this injury (see later: Fig. 5.48).

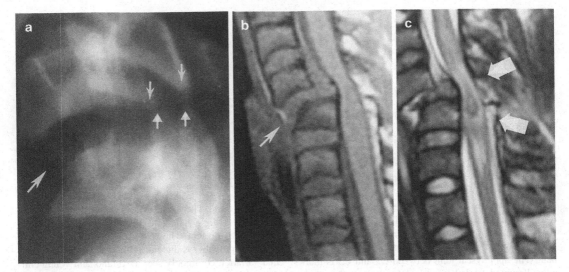

Fig. 5.9 Flexion force injuries: perched facette. (**a**) Note that the posterior inferior corners of both superior facettes (*upper posterior arrows*) are perched on the anterior superior corners of the lower vertebral body facettes (*lower posterior arrows*). The superior vertebral body is displaced on the inferior vertebral body, and there is minimal compression of the upper corner of the lower vertebral body (*anterior arrow*). (**b**) T1 sagittal MR study demonstrates the dislocated vertebral bodies (*arrow*) disrupted disk, some blood anterior to the vertebral bodies, and marked impingement of the spinal canal and cord. (**c**) T2 MR study demonstrates similar findings but more vividly demonstrates the cord contusion, small central hematoma, and edema around the fracture site (*arrows*)

Lateral Flexion Injuries

Pure lateral flexion injuries are uncommon, for this force usually is combined with some other force. Nonetheless, when compressive forces occur, they are present on the side of flexion, and distracting forces are present on the opposite side (Fig. 5.15). This results in compression of the vertebral body, fractures through the transverse processes on the side of flexion, and separation of the transverse processes, with ligamentous injuries along with avulsion fractures on the side of distraction. The dens also can be fractured and show lateral tilting.

Rotational Injuries

Rotational injuries usually are associated with anterior (flexion) or posterior (hyperextension) forces, but most often it is the former that occurs.

As a result, the superior facette of the involved joint is displaced anteriorly (Fig. 5.16). This finding is commonly seen on plain films, but it can be subtle (Fig. 5.17). The involved facette also can be perched or frankly locked over the inferior facette as with pure flexion injuries. On CT images, the disrupted apophyseal joint, along with surrounding fractures, is seen as the open facette sign (Fig. 5.18). Associated disk disruption secondary to ligamentous injury is common. As a result, the disk space frequently is narrowed and the superior vertebral body is displaced anteriorly on the inferior body. However, unless significant associated anterior compressive forces are present, there is no loss of height of the vertebral body (Fig. 5.18). Therefore, if one sees an anteriorly displaced vertebral body that appears to be intact and the disk space below it is narrowed, a rotational injury can be assumed. Other findings alerting one to the occurrence of a rotational injury are en face visualization of the pedicles

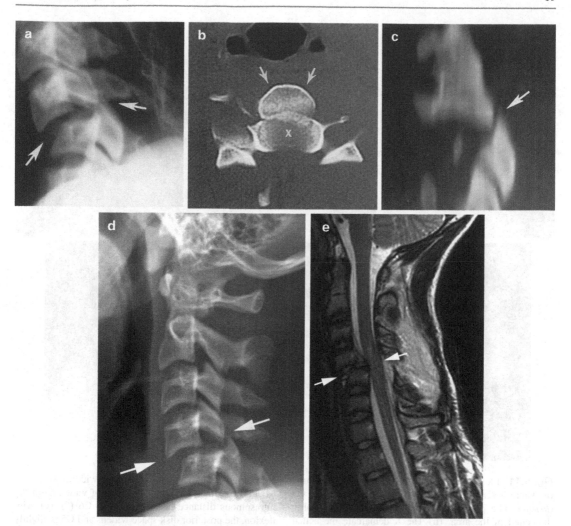

Fig. 5.10 Flexion force injuries: locked/jumped facettes. (**a**) The facettes are locked (*posterior arrow*), and there is complete dislocation of the vertebral bodies (*anterior arrow*). The involved intravertebral disk space is narrow. (**b**) On this axial CT image, the superior, dislocated vertebral body (*arrows*) is visible on the same plane as is the inferior vertebral body (X). Fractures of the lamina are present on the right. (**c**) Sagittal reconstructed CT study demonstrates the overlapping, "locked" facette (*arrow*). (**d**) Another patient. Note anterior dislocation of C4 on C5 (*anterior arrow*). The superior facette of the associated apophyseal joint has jumped over the inferior facette and is now locked (*posterior arrow*). (**e**) Sagittal T2 weighted MR study. Note the same dislocation as seen on plain films (*anterior arrow*). There also is posterior displacement (protrusion) in to the spinal canal with obliteration of the subarachnoid space and some compression of the spinal cord leading to mild contusion (*posterior arrow*). High signal edema is seen in the posterior soft tissues

above the level of rotation ("en face pedicle" sign) and narrowing of the space between the posterior cortex of the apophyseal joint and the anterior cortex of the spinous tip at levels above the injury (Fig. 5.17). Finally it should be noted that frequently both anterior flexion and anterior rotation forces are present. As a result, findings on the subsequent imaging studies can be mixed.

Posterior rotational injuries usually demonstrate little in the way of plain film findings. One may detect small avulsion fractures, and there may even be a fracture of the pars interarticularis on the side of rotation. The findings are similar to those seen with hyperextension injuries, and similarly the fractures are more readily demonstrable with computerized tomography.

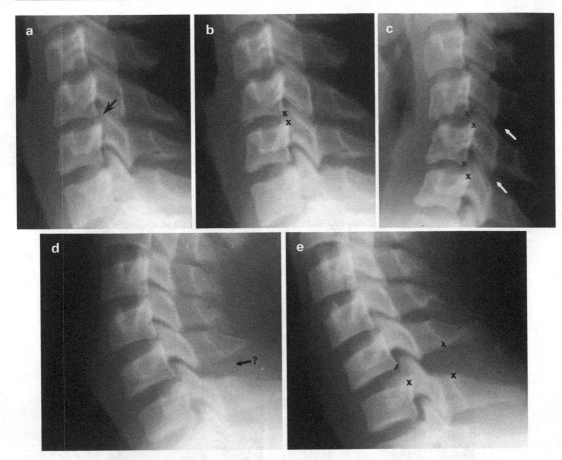

Fig. 5.11 Flexion force injury: occult ligament injury. (a) There is very slight anterior displacement of C4 on C5 (*arrow*). The prevertebral soft tissues are questionably thickened in the area. (b) The X demarcate the actual degree of slippage. (c) With flexion, there is now anterior displacement of C4 on C5 and C5 on C6 (X). The associ- ated apophyseal joints also are slightly widened (*arrows*). (d) In this patient there is suggestion of widening of the intraspinous distance between C5 and C6 (?). (e) With flexion, the posterior disk space widens and C5 is slightly anteriorly displaced on C6 (X). Posteriorly the intras- pinous distance becomes wider (X)

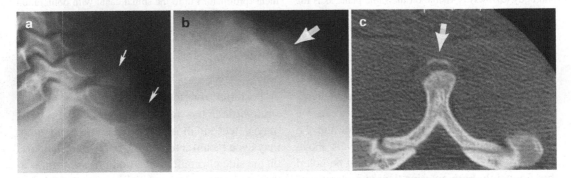

Fig. 5.12 Flexion force injury: spinous tip fracture. (a) Note spinous tip fractures of both C7 and T1 (*arrows*). (b) A very subtle spinous tip fracture (*arrow*). (c) CT study demonstrates the small bony fragment (*arrow*)

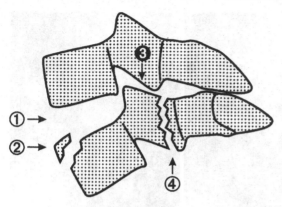

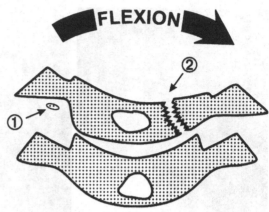

Fig. 5.13 Extension force injuries: diagrammatic representation. Note anterior disk widening (1), a teardrop fracture (2), disruption of the apophyseal joints (3), and a fracture through the pars (4)

Fig. 5.15 Lateral flexion force injuries: diagrammatic representation. With lateral flexion there often are avulsion fractures (1) on the diastatic side, while compression fractures (2) occur on the other side

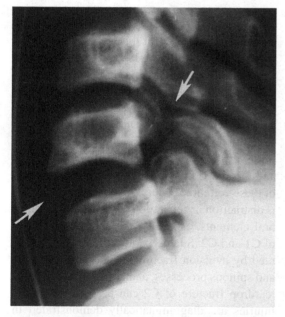

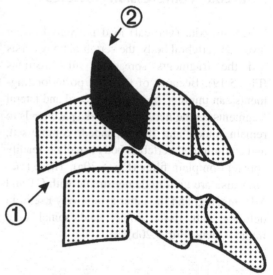

Fig. 5.14 Extension force injury: various findings. Note the widened disk space (*anterior arrow*) and slight anterior displacement of the superior vertebral body on the inferior vertebral body. Bilateral pars fractures are present (*posterior arrow*)

Fig. 5.16 Rotation force injuries: diagrammatic representation. Note anterior dislocation of the superior vertebral body and disk space narrowing (1). The superior facette is anteriorly displaced (2) because of rotation

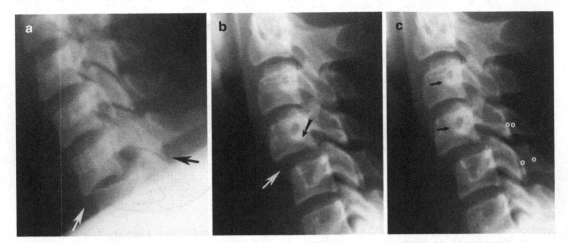

Fig. 5.17 Rotation force injuries: various plain findings. (**a**) Note the dislocated vertebral body and narrowed disk space (*white arrow*). No compression of the vertebral bodies is present. Posteriorly only one apophyseal joint is visualized (*black arrow*). Above this level, because the spine is rotated, two apophyseal joints are seen at each vertebral junction, one anterior to the other because of rotation. (**b**) In this patient there is vertebral body dislocation (*white arrow*). The disk space perhaps is slightly narrowed in comparison to the one above it. Also note that the superior facette is anteriorly displaced (*black arrow*) because of traumatic rotation. (**c**) Same patient demonstrating "en face" visualization of the pedicles (*black arrows*) above the level of rotation. In addition, posteriorly the distance between the apophyseal joint cortex and the cortex of the spinous tip is narrower above the level of rotation than below the level of rotation (Os)

Axial Load Compression Fractures

When an axial (vertical) load is exerted on an involved vertebral body, the vertebral body bursts and the fragments spread in all directions (Fig. 5.19). Because of this, the posterior fragments can impinge on the spinal cord and lateral fragments on the nerves. The disk space tends to remain intact, and the expanded, compressed, and comminuted vertebral body usually is readily apparent on plain films (Fig. 5.20a). These fractures also are vividly demonstrable with CT and MR imaging, and the latter also is very useful in defining soft tissue injury and spinal cord impingement (Fig. 5.20b).

Upper Cervical Spine (C1–C2) Injuries

Flexion Force Induced Injuries

When hyperflexion forces are applied to the upper cervical spine, although anterior compressive injuries might be expected, they are not common. The reason for this is structural for the first vertebra simply is a ring and the second vertebra a solid, tall pillar. This being the case, anterior compressive injuries cannot take their toll as they do on the rectangular vertebral bodies of the lower cervical vertebra. On the other hand, the same forces can easily overcome the protective limits of the posterior ligaments of C1 and C2, and C2 and C3. As a result anterior dislocation of these vertebrae occurs. At the same time, there is distraction or separation of the posterior vertebral elements, especially the spinous processes of C1 and C2. Such separation can be accompanied by avulsion fractures of the posterior arch and spinous processes, and occasionally anterior teardrop fracture of C2 can be seen. All these injuries are diagrammatically demonstrated in Fig. 5.21.

In terms of anterior compression induced fractures of C1 and C2, although rare, vertical fractures of the anterior arch of C1 [25] and hyperflexion-induced avulsion (teardrop) fractures of the lower anterior corner of the body of C2 are sometimes encountered (Fig. 5.22a, b).

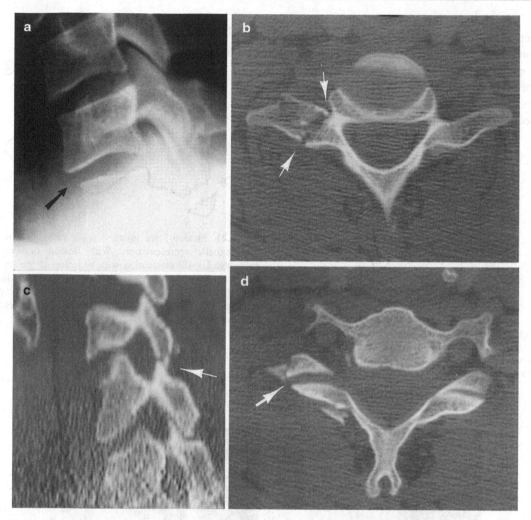

Fig. 5.18 Rotation force injury: plain film and CT findings. (**a**) Note the narrowed vertebral disk space and slight anterior dislocation of the superior vertebral body (*arrow*). (**b**) Axial CT study of the lower vertebra demonstrates a fracture (*arrows*) through the pars. (**c**) At a slightly higher level, the "open facette" sign (*arrow*) of the dislocated apophyseal joint is seen. Scattered fractures are seen in the area. (**d**) Sagittal reconstruction CT study demonstrates a "perched facette" on the side of dislocation (*arrow*). Small bony fracture fragments are seen in the area

Overall, hyperflexion forces more often are dissipated through the C1–C2 ligaments, with resultant anterior dislocation of C1 on C2. Radiographically this results in widening of the predental distance and increase in the interspinous distance (Fig. 5.22c).

Anteriorly angled or frankly displaced dens fractures also can result from hyperflexion injuries, and are common. In infants and young children, such fractures usually occur through the dens body synchondrosis (Fig. 5.23). Although this location is most common in infants and young children [8, 9, 26], it should be noted that similar fractures can occur at the os terminale–dens synchondrosis. In such cases the os terminale can be anteriorly dislocated on the dens, and often there is resultant posttraumatic resorption of the dens, overgrowth of the os terminale, and the development of an acquired os odontoideum, as shown earlier (see Fig. 4.14).

In older children and adolescents, once the dens body synchondrosis has fused, dens fractures tend to resemble those seen in the adult population. Most of these fractures occur through the base of the dens and can be subtle (Figs. 5.24 and 5.25). Fractures also can occur through the body or the tip of the dens.

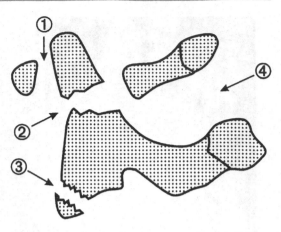

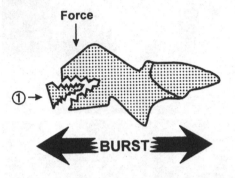

Fig. 5.19 Axial compressive force injuries: diagrammatic representation. Upon application of axial force (Force), the vertebral body bursts, and fragments are disbursed in various outward directions (1)

Fig. 5.21 Flexion force injuries: upper cervical spine; diagrammatic representation. With flexion one can encounter C1–C2 dislocation with widening of the predental distance (1), fractures through the dens, usually through the base (2), and occasionally anterior teardrop fractures (3). Posteriorly the intraspinous distance can increase (4)

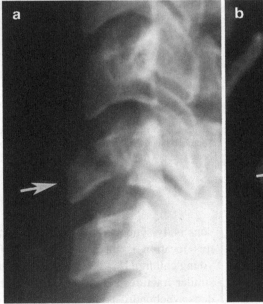

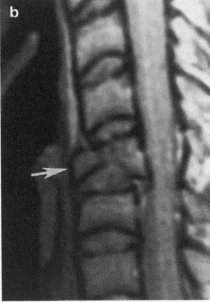

Fig. 5.20 Axial compressive force injuries. (**a**) Note the compressed, fragmented, and expanded vertebral body (*arrow*). (**b**) A subsequent MR sagittal view demonstrates the expanded vertebral body (*arrow*) protruding anteriorly into the soft tissues and posteriorly into the spinal canal causing some cord compression

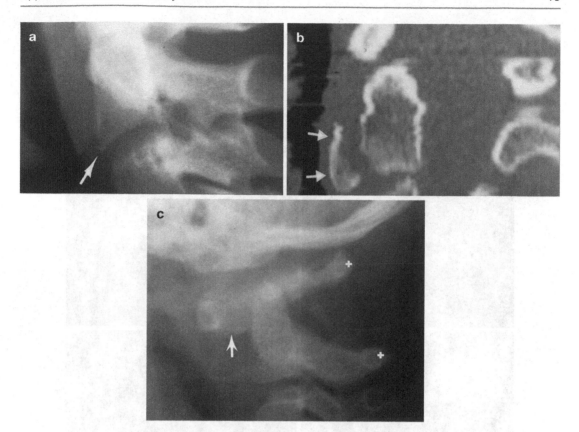

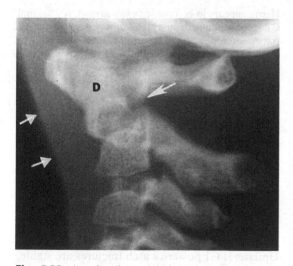

Fig. 5.22 Flexion force injuries: various types. (**a**) Note the small avulsion–teardrop fracture of C2 (*arrow*). The prevertebral soft tissues are borderline in suggesting swelling. (**b**) Another patient with a large avulsion teardrop fracture (*arrows*). (**c**) In this patient there is frank dislocation of C1 and C2 with marked increase in the predental distance (*anterior arrow*). This is associated with a marked increase in the intraspinous distance posteriorly (+)

Fig. 5.23 Anterior force injuries: dens fractures in infants. Note the anteriorly tilted dens (D). The fracture has occurred through the dens–body synchondrosis (*posterior arrow*). The dens is displaced forward on the body of C2. There is considerable prevertebral soft tissue swelling (*anterior arrows*)

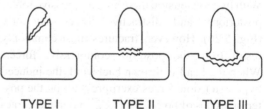

TYPE I   TYPE II   TYPE III

Fig. 5.24 Dens fractures in older children: classification. The types of fractures occurring in older children is the same as in adults. The type II and III fractures are most unstable

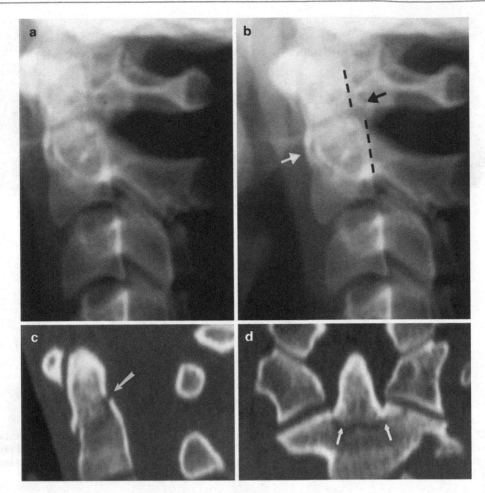

Fig. 5.25 Anterior force injury: dens fracture in older child. (**a**) The findings are very subtle. Can you appreciate them? (**b**) Same patient, demonstrating that the dens is anteriorly displaced on the body of C2 (*black arrow* and *dashed lines*). The anterior cortex of the ring of Harris appears to be double (*white arrow*). (**c**) Sagittal CT reconstruction demonstrates an anteriorly displaced fracture through the base of the dens (*arrow*). (**d**) Coronal reconstruction demonstrates the same fracture (*arrows*)

Hyperextension Force Induced Injuries

With hyperextension there are compressive forces posteriorly and distractive forces anteriorly (Fig. 5.26). However, fractures most commonly result from the posterior compressive forces. When the head is thrown backward, the induced hyperextension forces exert pressure on the posterior arches of both C1 and C2, and indeed, fractures of the posterior arches of both C1 and C2 both are common.

Fractures occurring through the posterior arch of C1 manifest in thin, radiolucent bony defects (Fig. 5.27). The edges of these defects do not show sclerosis and thus are readily differentiated from the much more common bizarre array of posterior C1 congenital defects considered in Chap. 3 (see Figs. 3.16 and 3.17). Unilateral C1 posterior arch fractures are stable, and indeed, bilateral posterior C1 neural arch fractures probably also are stable as long as they are not associated with other injuries, which might convert the overall injury into one that is unstable.

When C2 is involved in a hyperextension-induced injury, fracturing of the neural arch, usually through the area of the pars intra-articularis

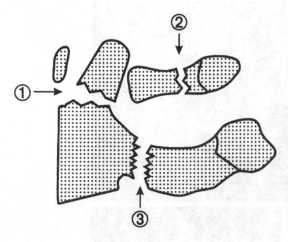

Fig. 5.26 Extension force injuries: diagrammatic representation. Hyperextension injuries can lead to posteriorly displaced and posteriorly tilted dens fractures (1), vertical fractures through the neural arch of C1 (2), and similar fractures through the pars of C2 (3)

occurs, constituting the typical *hangman's fracture of C2* (Figs. 5.28 and 5.29). The mechanism of injury is the same as that which exists at the C1 level, for with hyperextension forces there is posterior dissipation of compressive forces through the neural arches. Hangman's fractures may be difficult to see on lateral radiographs of the cervical spine, but in other cases, diastasis of the fracture is more clearly visible (Fig. 5.28). In the more occult cases, use of the posterior cervical line [27] can be helpful. The reason for this is that very often there is associated anterior displacement (dislocation) of C2 on C3 and such dislocation must be differentiated from normal subluxation of C2 on C3 (see Fig. 2.11). *With hangman's fractures, the posterior cervical line, when applied from the anterior cortex of the spinous tip of C1 to the anterior cortex of the spinous tip of C3, misses the anterior cortex of the spinous tip of C2 by 1.5 mm or more* (Fig. 5.29). When bilateral fractures occur through the pars intra-articularis or the neural arches, instability is inevitable. However, if these fractures occur unilaterally, they are not unstable

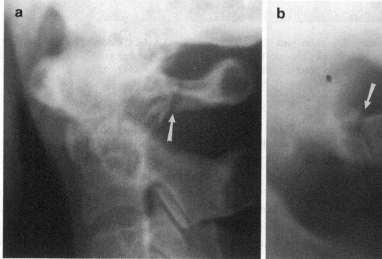

Fig. 5.27 Hyperextension posterior C1 fractures. (**a**) Note the thin, radiolucent line (*arrow*) representing a posterior neural arch fracture. In this patient the dens also was fractured. Though difficult to see, the ring of Harris is disrupted. (**b**) Tomogram more clearly demonstrates the radiolucent fracture defect (*arrow*), without sclerotic edges

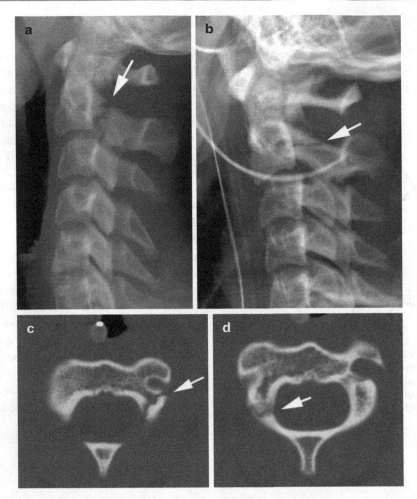

Fig. 5.28 Hangman's fracture: plain film and CT findings. (**a**) Note the clearly visible fracture through the neural arch of C2 (*arrow*). C2 is slightly anteriorly displaced on C3. (**b**) In this patient the fracture is visible but less distinct. (**c**) Axial CT demonstrates a clear-cut fracture (*arrow*). (**d**) Another axial CT slice demonstrates a fracture on the other side (*arrow*)

(Fig. 5.30), and finally it is important to appreciate that while much attention is devoted to the typical hangman's fracture of C2, fractures in this area can be more complex. In addition, because hyperextension and hyperflexion forces are both present in some patients, features of both hyperflexion and hyperextension induces injuries will be seen (Figs. 5.31 and 5.32).

With hyperextension forces, although distraction forces are present anteriorly, injuries secondary to such forces are less common than in the lower cervical spine. Occasionally one can sustain anterior C1 arch avulsion fractures, and anterior avulsion fractures of the body of C2. In addition, in some cases one will see anterior widening of the disk space between C2 and C3 (Fig. 5.31). Hyperextension forces also lead to posteriorly displaced or tilted dens fractures (Figs. 5.33 and 5.34). In some cases findings suggest mixed hyperextension/flexion forces, that is a whiplash injury (Fig. 5.35). Finally, the posteriorly tilted and displaced dens must be

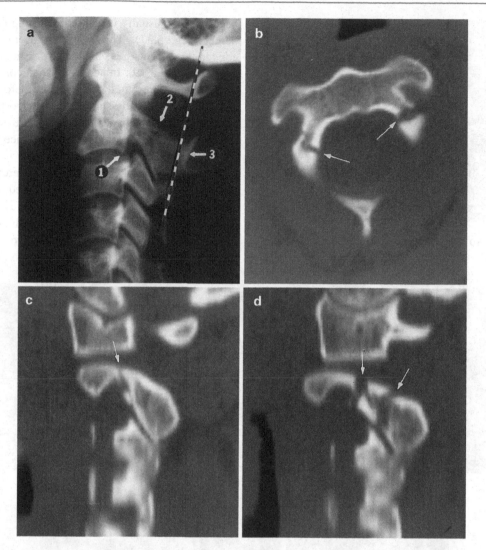

Fig. 5.29 Extension force injury: hangman fracture with posterior cervical line applied. (**a**) Note anterior displacement of C2 on C3 (1). A subtle fracture through the pars is suggested (2), and the posterior cervical line (*dashed line*) is abnormal, missing the posterior cortex of the spinous tip of C2 by 2 mm (3). (**b**) Axial CT study demonstrates bilateral pars fractures (*arrows*). (**c**) Sagittal reconstruction on one side demonstrates a pars fracture (*arrow*). (**d**) On the other side a comminuted pars fracture is seen (*arrows*)

differentiated from the more frequently encountered normal posteriorly tilted dens shown earlier (see Fig. 4.17).

Hyperextension injuries leading to hangman's fractures in infants can pose a problem in terms of differentiating the resultant bony defect from congenital defects that can occur at this site. Moreover, these fractures can be relatively silent,

further complicating the problem [28]. These fractures also have been documented in the battered child syndrome [28–30].

To differentiate a fracture from a congenital defect, it should be remembered that with a hangman's fracture there is no sclerosis of the edges of the bony defect (Fig. 5.36). Furthermore, with flexion, considerable instability will be apparent

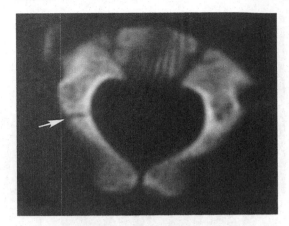

Fig. 5.30 Extension force injury: unilateral pars fracture. Note the unilateral, nondisplaced pars fracture (*arrow*)

because there usually is marked widening of the defect (Fig. 5.37). This does not occur with congenital defects, as illustrated earlier (see Figs. 3.18 and 3.19). In addition, when congenital defects are present, the edges of the defect are sclerotic and relatively smooth, and the posterior arch of C2 along with adjacent arches are underdeveloped and anomalous in appearance (see Fig. 3.19).

Finally it should be recalled that hyperextension injuries of the upper cervical spine frequently are seen in association with facial injuries [31]. The same now has been documented with airbag injuries [32] and this is very important, for often the facial injuries in both situations are so exten-

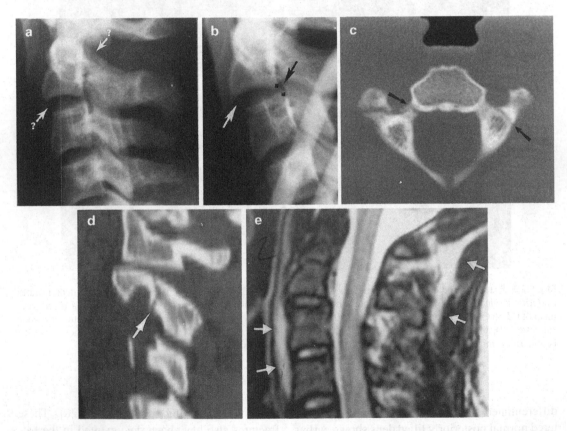

Fig. 5.31 Extension force injury: hangman's fracture with C2–C3 disk disruption. (**a**) There is subtle suggestion of a pars fracture (*upper arrow with question mark*). In addition the anterior C2–C3 disk space suggests widening (*lower arrow with question mark*). (**b**) Later, the fracture is more difficult to see, but anterior disk space widening is more clearly identified (*white arrow*), and now there is anterior displacement of C2 on C3 (*posterior arrow and squares*). (**c**) Axial CT demonstrates bilateral pars fractures (*arrows*). (**d**) Sagittal reconstruction on one side demonstrates a nondisplaced pars fracture (*arrow*). A similar fracture was present on the other side. (**e**) Sagittal MR study demonstrates anterior and posterior soft tissue edema (*arrows*) secondary to ligament damage, C2 is slightly anteriorly displaced on C3. The spinal cord is normal. Increased signal is due to flow artifact. In this patient the overall findings suggest both flexion and extension forces; that is a whiplash injury

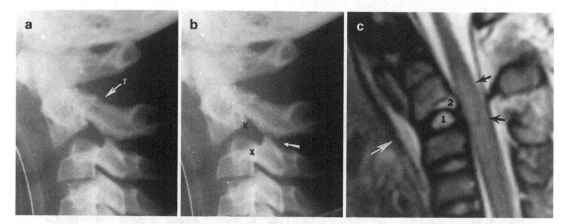

Fig. 5.32 Extension–flexion (mixed) force injury: hangman's fracture with disk disruption. (**a**) Note suggestion of a hangman's fracture (*arrow with question mark*). (**b**) Also note that the posterior disk space at C2–C3 is markedly increased (X). The associated apophyseal joint is V-shaped, and sprung in configuration (*arrow*). (**c**) Sagittal MR T2 study demonstrates anterior edema (*anterior arrow*), bulging of the disk (1) and a fracture fragment (2), all of which protrude into the spinal canal, obliterating the subarachnoid space. The spinal cord demonstrates associated swelling and contusion (*black arrows*). In this patient the resulting injury suggests both flexion and extension forces; that is a whiplash injury

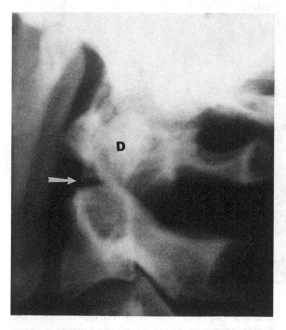

Fig. 5.33 Extension force injury: posteriorly tilted dens. The dens (D) is posteriorly tilted. A fracture through the base (*arrow*) is present. The prevertebral soft tissues are prominent

sive that they distract one's attention from the cervical spine. However, the underlying cervical spine injury may be even more life-threatening.

Lateral Flexion Force Induced Injuries

Pure lateral flexion injuries of the upper cervical spine are rather uncommon. They can result in fractures through the base of the dens, with lateral dens tilting (Fig. 5.38). In addition, compression injuries involving the side towards which flexion occurs can be seen. At the same time, avulsion injuries involving the contralateral vertebral bodies and arches can occur. However, as noted, these injuries in pure form are rather uncommon. Most often lateral flexion injuries are associated with some other force.

Rotational Force Induced Injuries

Rotational injuries of C1 on C2 are common [33, 34], and anterior rotational injuries are more common than posterior rotational injuries. In this regard, with anterior rotation injuries of C1 on C2, the involved lateral mass of C1 comes to lie in front of the lateral mass and body of C2 (Fig. 5.39) and with frank dislocation, a most peculiar posture of the head on the neck is assumed. In such cases, while the cervical spine below the level of C1 is sagittal in orientation, C1

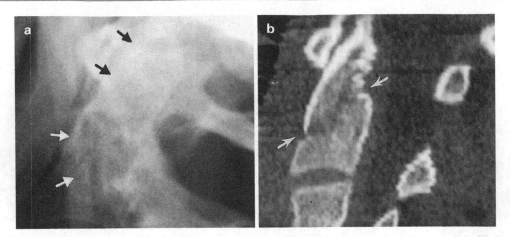

Fig. 5.34 Extension force injuries: subtle dens fracture. (**a**) The dens (*black arrows*) is posteriorly tilted. However, no clear-cut fracture is seen but the ring of Harris (*white arrows*) is not clearly visible and appears to be disrupted. (**b**) Sagittal tomogram demonstrates a fracture through the base of the dens (*arrows*)

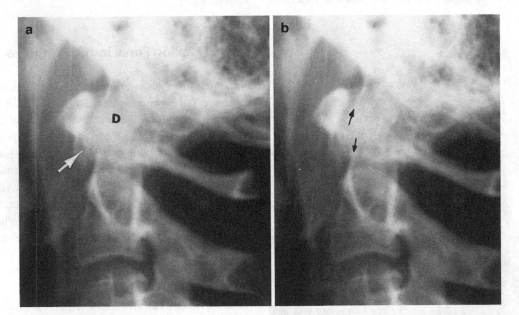

Fig. 5.35 Extension force injury: posteriorly tilted dens. (**a**) Note that the posteriorly tilted dens (D) is also anteriorly displaced (*arrow*) through the base. (**b**) Anterior displacement is defined by the arrows overlying the anterior cortices of the dens and body of C2. Most likely both hyperextension and flexion forces were applied (i.e., whiplash injury)

and the skull are rotated 90° and are oriented in coronal projection (Fig. 5.39d). Although the findings are very dramatic and troublesome, the neck is stable within this configuration. Treatment in all these cases usually consists of administration of muscle relaxants [34].

In many cases the predental distance increases, but this does not always happen. When C2 is

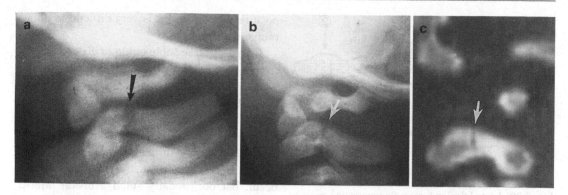

Fig. 5.36 Extension force injury: hangman's fracture in infants. (**a**) Note the typical hangman's fracture (*arrow*) in this infant. There are no sclerotic edges to the fracture. The spinous process of C2 is normally developed. (**b**) A more subtle fracture (*arrow*) is present in this infant. Note that the neural arch of C2 is normally formed. (**c**) Sagittal reconstructed CT study demonstrates the same fracture (*arrow*)

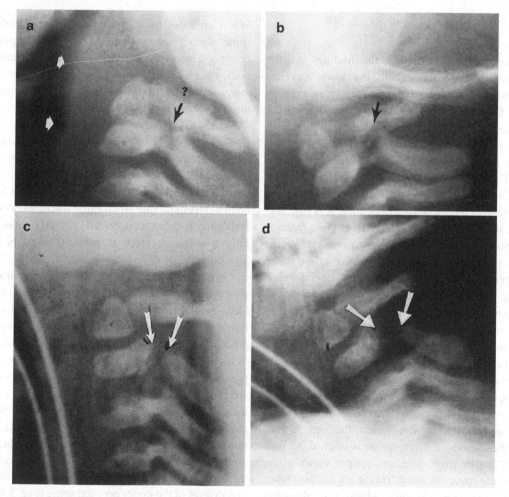

Fig. 5.37 Extension force injury: value of flexion view in identifying hangman's fracture in infants. (**a**) A fracture is barely suggested (*black arrow*). However, the prevertebral soft tissues (*white arrows*) are thickened. (**b**) With flexion there is marked widening of the fracture line (*arrow*). (**c**) In this patient a clearly visible hangman's fracture is present (*arrows*). (**d**) With flexion there is marked widening of the fracture space (*arrows*)

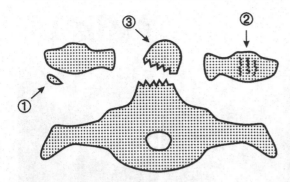

Fig. 5.38 Lateral flexion forces: diagrammatic representation of injuries. Patients may sustain, on the diastatic side, avulsion fractures (1) and on the compressive side, fractures of the arch of C1 (2) One can also encounter laterally tilted dens fractures (3)

anteriorly rotated on C3, the findings are the same as those throughout the lower cervical spine. There are varying degrees of severity of C1–C2 rotational injuries, the mildest being the so called "wry neck." In this condition there usually is no history of trauma. The usual scenario is that the patient awakens in the morning, has a stiff neck, and cannot turn it to one side or the other. The condition is self-limiting and probably represents a mild degree of subluxation with secondary muscle spasm. The radiographic findings consist of tilting of the head to one side or the other on the AP view and flexion–rotation of the upper cervical spine on the lateral view (Fig. 5.40). On frontal view, if a line is drawn down the midaxis of the dens, both the apex of the mandibular angle and the spinous tip of C2 lie to the same side of the line (Fig. 5.40c). This is the opposite of what occurs when simple rotation is present. With simple rotation, the spinous tip of C2 and the apex of the mandibular angle lie on opposite sides of the vertical line drawn through the midsagittal plane of the dens. In most of these cases, muscle spasm is intense but usually can be overcome, and proper views of the cervical spine obtained. This is not the case when true dislocation occurs where the abnormal

position is fixed and it is very difficult to obtain proper radiographs.

In cases of true subluxation or dislocation, the fixed nature of the injury can be demonstrated with dynamic CT imaging [34]. With this study one will be able to see, very clearly, that while normal motion occurs when the head is turned to the normal side, there is fixation of C1 on C2 when the head is turned to the abnormal side (Fig. 5.41). In most of these cases no fractures occur, but occasionally small avulsion injuries are encountered.

Axial Force Induced Injuries

When an axial load is applied to the cervical spine, forces are dissipated through the spinal column. However, since the first two vertebral bodies act as shock absorbers for such injuries, many more pure axial loading, exploding fractures involve these two vertebra (Fig. 5.42).

When C1 is involved, the term "Jefferson fracture" is applied. The number of fractures present is variable and can range from a single fracture in one of the arches to four fractures, two on each side. In terms of instability, it has been determined that when three fractures occur, instability is most pronounced [35]. Of course, if only a single fracture is present, there is no instability.

On plain films there usually is very little to see on the lateral view with Jefferson (C1) fractures. Occasionally one can see upper prevertebral soft tissue swelling (Fig. 5.43a), but such swelling is difficult to differentiate from normal prominence of the soft tissues in this area. Because of this, the presence or absence of prevertebral soft tissue swelling is of little value in analyzing these cases. Initial diagnosis, therefore, rests on the open-mouth odontoid view. On this view the lateral masses, or mass of C1, will be laterally displaced on the lateral masses or mass of C2. To be valid, the finding should be present on true AP (no rotation) views of the upper cervical spine (Fig. 5.43).

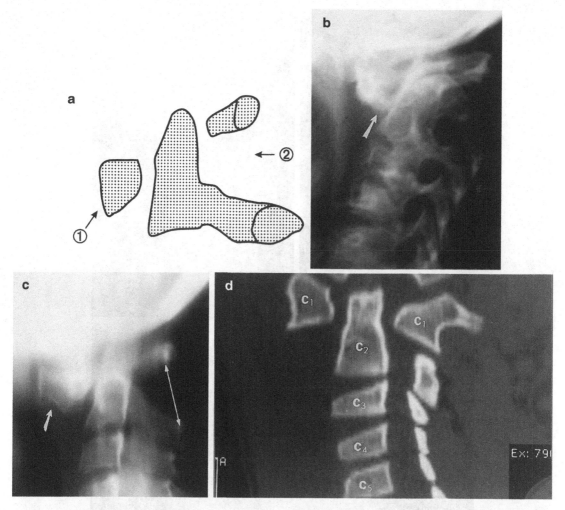

Fig. 5.39 Rotational force injuries: C1–C2 rotatory dislocation. (**a**) Diagrammatic representation. As C1 rotates on C2, the anterior arch of C1 is dislocated anteriorly (1) and the predental distance increases. At the same time, there is an increase in the intraspinous distance between C1 and C2 posteriorly (2). (**b**) Lateral view demonstrates a totally distorted upper cervical spine and a wide predental distance (*arrow*). The C1–C2 intraspinous distance is also increased but is difficult to visualize. (**c**) Tomogram demonstrates the anteriorly displaced lateral mass of C1 (*anterior arrow*). In addition, now the increase in the intraspinous distance between C1 and C2 is clearly evident (*posterior arrows* and *line*). (**d**) In this patient the cervical spine from C2–C5 is visualized in the sagittal plane, but C1, because it is rotated is displayed in the coronal plane

This is important because it is well known that with rotation, and indeed, even without rotation, in normal individuals, the lateral masses can appear laterally displaced. The latter is especially likely to occur in early infancy, where as noted earlier the finding most often is normal (see Fig. 2.28). All this can be further aggravated by the ever-present hypermobility of the childhood spine secondary to normal ligament laxity (see Fig. 2.29). In the end, Jefferson fractures are most vividly delineated with axial CT views (Fig. 5.44).

When C2 fractures result from axial loading forces, the bursting phenomenon generally occurs through the body and not the dens of C2.

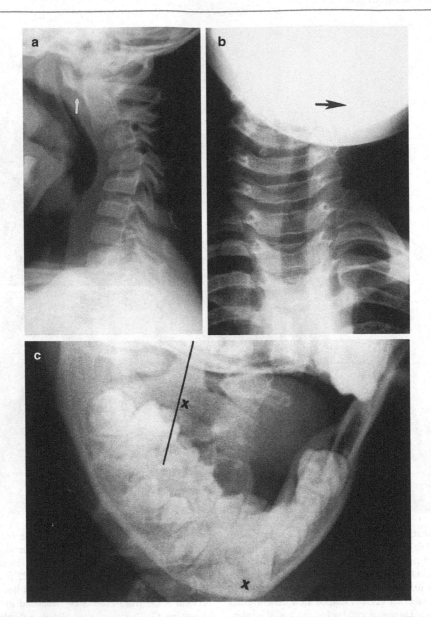

Fig. 5.40 Rotation force injury: wry neck. (**a**) Note marked kyphosis and rotation of the cervical spine. The predental distance (*arrow*) still is normal and the prevertebral soft tissues are normal. (**b**) The AP view demonstrates deviation of the head and chin to the left (*arrow*). (**c**) The point of measurement is indicated by the line drawn down the mid axis of the dens. The spinous tip of C2 (*upper* X) and the tip of the mandible (*lower* X) lie to the same side of the line drawn through the mid-longitudinal axis of the dens (i.e., to the side of rotation). Normally they would lie on opposite sides of the line

The posterior arch, as opposed to the posterior arch of C1, is seldom involved. On plain lateral films the body of C2 appears unusually wide and hence the "fat" C2 sign [36]. Occasionally the body of C2 can normally appear rather wide; if the body of C2 appears fat when trauma is present, however, one should suspect a bursting fracture (Fig. 5.45) and proceed to CT imaging.

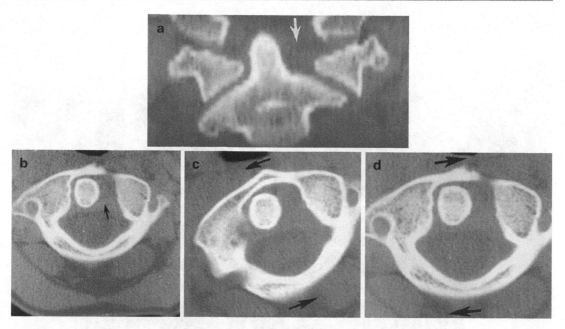

Fig. 5.41 Rotatory force injury: fixation-use of dynamic CT. (**a**) Coronal reconstruction demonstrates a wide left lateral mass–dens distance (*arrow*). The left lateral mass is offset. (**b**) Axial CT demonstrates the wide left lateral mass–dens distance (*arrow*). (**c**) With rotation to the right C1 rotates to the right (*arrows*). (**d**) With rotation to the left, C1 cannot rotate because it is fixed in the midline (*arrows*)

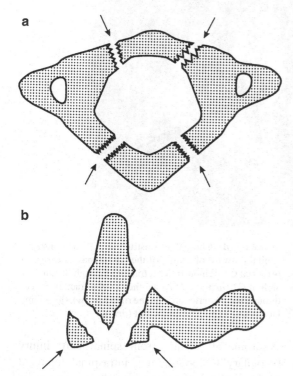

Fig. 5.42 Axial compression force injury: diagrammatic representation. (**a**) Note fractures through four sites (*arrows*) of the ring of C1. (**b**) Compression axial loading on C2 produces a burst or "fat" vertebra (*arrows*)

Atlanto-Occipital Disassociation

Complete disruption of the ligaments between the cervical spine and occiput occurs with severe trauma [37–39]. Most often the patient has been involved in a motor vehicle accident. In severe cases, the problem is not difficult to detect on plain films (Fig. 5.46a). On the other hand, in more subtle cases it may be difficult to distinguish the findings from those seen in some normal individuals. Some normal individuals have a deceptively wide atlanto-occipital distance. To aid in deciphering this dilemma, it has been demonstrated that when both the basion–axial distance and basion–dental distance are 12 mm or less the distance between the occiput and C1 can be considered normal [40]. However, in children less than 13 years old, these figures are less reliable [40]. Therefore, the evaluation of the radiographs in children remains somewhat subjective (Fig. 5.46).

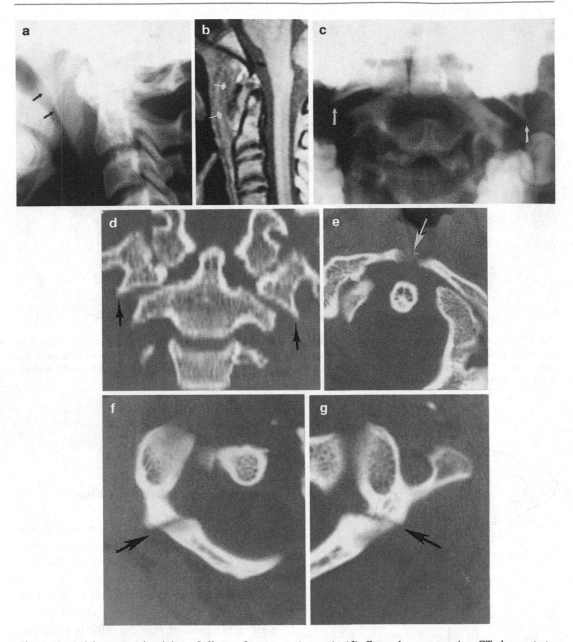

Fig. 5.43 Axial compression injury: Jefferson fracture. (a) Note some prevertebral soft tissue swelling (*arrows*). This is uncommonly seen with Jefferson fractures. (b) This MR T2 study demonstrates edema and bleeding anterior to C1 and the dens (*arrows*). (c) Open-mouth odontoid view demonstrates bilateral offset lateral masses (*arrows*). (d) Coronal reconstruction CT demonstrates similar outward offsetting of the lateral masses (*arrows*). (e) Axial CT demonstrates a fracture through the anterior arch of C1 (*arrow*). (f) At another level a fracture is seen through the posterior arch on the right (*arrow*). (g) A similar fracture is present on the left (*arrow*)

SCIWORA Syndrome

The SCIWORA syndrome, representing spinal cord injury without radiographic findings [23, 24], was formerly known as the central cord syndrome. It results from spinal cord injury secondary to longitudinal, intraspinal ligament buckling with hyperextension. There are no plain film findings, but clinical findings will suggest a neurologic deficit at the mid- to lower cervical

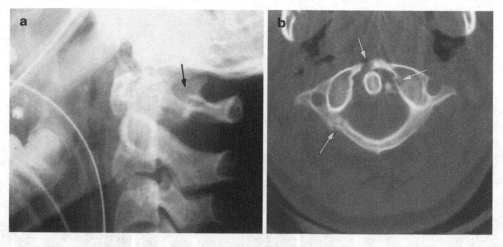

Fig. 5.44 Axial compression injury: Jefferson fracture. (a) The upper cervical spine is normal. The apparently offset arch of C1 (*arrow*) should not be misinterpreted for a fracture. It is a normal artifact (see Fig. 2.26). (b) Same patient demonstrating fractures through three sites (*arrows*) of the ring of C1

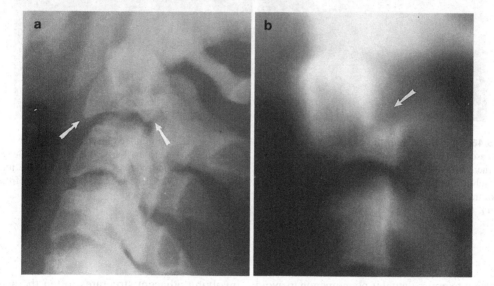

Fig. 5.45 Axial compression injury: "fat" C2. (a) Although a fracture is not seen, the body of C2 is unusually wide (*arrows*) and hence the "fat" C2 sign. (b) Tomogram demonstrates the bursting fracture of the dens (*arrow*)

cord level. Magnetic resonance imaging is required for demonstration of the contusion or hemorrhage sustained in these injuries (Fig. 5.47).

Brachial Plexus Injuries

Brachial plexus injuries result from lateral flexion, and stretching injuries apply to the cervical spine. There are no plain film findings unless associated fractures are seen. Again, while in the past brachial plexus nerve injuries were demonstrated with myelography, now they are routinely demonstrable with MR imaging (Fig. 5.48).

Motion Artifact: Pseudofracture CT Reconstruction

With CT reconstruction, motion always is a problem. Such motion can produce artifacts that suggest vertebral fractures (Fig. 5.49). It is most

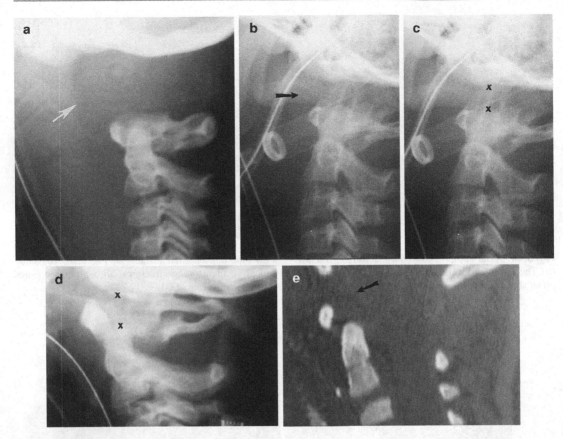

Fig. 5.46 Atlanto-occipital disassociation. (**a**) In this gross case, the space between the occiput and C1 is markedly increased (*arrow*). (**b**) This patient demonstrates more subtle findings, but still the distance between the base of the skull and C1 along with the dens is prominent (*arrow*). (**c**) The dens–basion distance (X) is increased and measures 13 mm. (**d**) Another patient with subtle findings. The dens–basion distance (X) is increased. (**e**) Sagittal reconstruction CT demonstrates the findings more clearly. The dens is markedly separated from the base of the skull (*arrow*)

important to appreciate this phenomenon to avoid misinterpreting the findings as indicating a fracture. To aid in this differentiation, one should look for similar irregularities, on the same plane, involving adjacent structures, often the airway. If there is irregularity and offsetting of the airway at the same level, a motion artifact should be suspected.

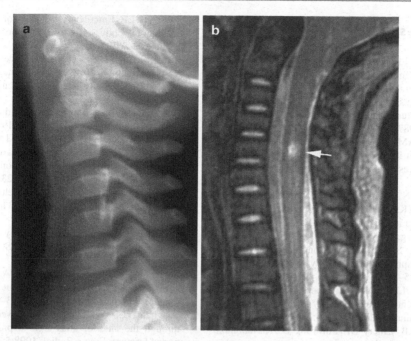

Fig. 5.47 Cord contusion: "SCIWORA" syndrome. (**a**) In this patient with cord symptoms the cervical spine is completely normal. (**b**) Sagittal MR, T2 weighted demonstrates swelling of the upper cord and a focal area of high signal/contusion (*arrows*)

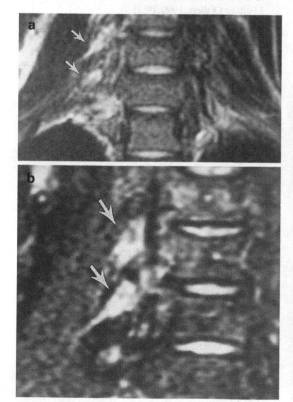

Fig. 5.48 Brachial plexus injury. (**a**) Note the altered nerve roots on the right (*arrows*). (**b**) Fat suppression study demonstrates the cerebrospinal fluid (CSF) surrounding the nerve routes more clearly (*arrows*)

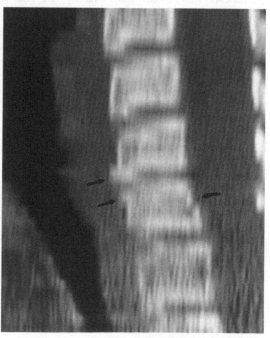

Fig. 5.49 Motion artifact: pseudofractures. On reconstructed views, patient motion often leads to artifacts that closely mimic fractures (*arrows*)

References

1. Swischuk LE, Swischuk PN, John SD. Wedging of C–3 in infants and children: usually a normal finding and not a fracture. Radiology. 1993;188:523–6.
2. Apple JS, Kirks DR, Merten DF, Martinez S. Cervical spine fractures and dislocations in children. Pediatr Radiol. 1987;17:45–9.
3. Dietrich AM, Ginn-Pease ME, Barkowski HM, King DR. Pediatric cervical spine fractures: predominantly subtle presentation. J Pediatr Surg. 1991;26: 995–1000.
4. Hadley MN, Babramski JM, Browner CM, Rekate H, Sonntag VKH. Pediatric spinal trauma: review of 122 cases of spinal cord and vertebral column injuries. J Neurosurg. 1988;68:18–24.
5. Ruge JR, Sinson GP, McLone DG, Cerullo LJ. Pediatric spinal injury: the very young. J Neurosurg. 1988;68:25–30.
6. Swischuk LE, John SD, Hendrick EP. Is the open mouth odontoid view necessary in children under five years? Pediatr Radiol. 2000;30:186–9.
7. Connolly B, Emery D, Armstrong D. The odontoid synchondrotic slip: an injury unique to young children. Pediatr Radiol. 1995;25:S129–33.
8. Griffiths SC. Fracture of odontoid process in children. J Pediatr Surg. 1972;7:680–3.
9. Sherk HH, Nicholson JT, Chung SMK. Fractures of the odontoid process in young children. J Bone Joint Surg Am. 1978;60A:921–4.
10. Blacksin MF, Lee HJ. Frequency and significance of fractures of the upper cervical spine detected by CT in patients with severe head trauma. AJR Am J Roentgenol. 1995;165:1201–4.
11. Bloom AI, Neeman Z, Floman Y, Gomori J, Bar-Ziv J. Occipital condyle fracture and ligament injury: imaging by CT. Pediatr Radiol. 1996;26:786–90.
12. Nunez Jr DB, Quencer RM. The role of helical CT in the assessment of cervical spine injuries. AJR Am J Roentgenol. 1988;171:951–7.
13. Poirier VC, Greenlaw AR, Beatty CS, Seibert JA, Abliun DS. Computed tomographic evaluation of C1–C2 in pediatric cervical spine trauma. Emerg Radiol. 1994;1:195–9.
14. Orenstein JB, Klein BI, Ochenschlager DW. Delayed diagnosis of pediatric cervical spine injury. Pediatrics. 1992;89:1185–8.
15. Woods WA, Brady WJ, Pollock G, Kini N, Young JS. Flexion–extension cervical spine radiography in pediatric blunt trauma. Emerg Radiol. 1998;5:381–4.
16. Dwek JR, Chung CB. Radiography of cervical spine injury in children: are flexion–extension radiographs useful for acute trauma? AJR Am J Roentgenol. 2000;174:1617–9.
17. Clark WM, Gehweiler Jr JA, Laib R. Twelve significant signs of cervical spine trauma. Skeletal Radiol. 1979;3:201–5.
18. Swischuk LE. Emergency radiology of the acutely ill or injured child. 4th ed. Baltimore: Lippincott Williams & Wilkins; 2000. p. 546.
19. Kim KS, Chen HH, Russell EJ, Rogers LF. Flexion teardrop fracture of the cervical spine: radiographic characteristics. AJR Am J Roentgenol. 1989;152: 319–26.
20. Gooding CA, Hurwitz ME. Avulsed vertebral rim apophysis in a child. Pediatr Radiol. 1974;2:265–8.
21. Naidich JB, Naidich TP, Garfein C, Liebeskind AL, Hyman RA. The widened interspinous distance: a useful sign of anterior cervical dislocation in the supine frontal projection. Radiology. 1977;123:113–6.
22. Cintron E, Gilula IA, Murphy WA, Gehweiler JA. The widened disk space: a sign of cervical hyperextension injury. Radiology. 1981;141:639–44.
23. Pang D, Pollack IF. Spinal cord injury without radiographic abnormality in children: the SCIWORA syndrome. J Trauma. 1989;29:654–64.
24. Ingve DA, Harris WP, Herndon WA, Sullivan JA, Gross RH. Spinal cord injury without osseous spine fracture. J Pediatr Orthop. 1988;8:153–9.
25. Vaughan TE, West OC. Isolated vertical fracture through the anterior atlas arch: a previously unreported fracture. Emerg Radiol. 1998;5:259–62.
26. Odent T, Langlais J, Clorion C, Kassis B, Bataille J, Pouliquen JC. Fractures of the odontoid process: a report of 15 cases in children younger than six years. J Pediatr Orthop. 1999;19:51–4.
27. Swischuk LE. Anterior displacement of C2 in children: physiologic or pathologic? A helpful differentiation. Radiology. 1977;122:759–63.
28. Kleinman PK, Shelton YA. Hangman's fracture in an abused infant: imaging features. Pediatr Radiol. 1997;27:776–7.
29. McGrory BE, Fenichel GM. Hangman's fracture subsequent to shaking an infant. Ann Neurol. 1977;2:82.
30. Weiss MH, Kaufman B. Hangman's fracture in an infant. Am J Dis Child. 1973;126:268–9.
31. Haug RH, Wible RT, Likavec MJ, Conforti PJ. Cervical spine fractures and maxillofacial trauma. J Oral Maxillofac Surg. 1991;49:725–9.
32. Gigeure JF, St-Vil D, Turmel A, et al. Airbags and children; a spectrum of C-spine injuries. J Pediatr Surg. 1998;33:811–6.
33. Muniz AE, Belfer RA. Atlantoaxial rotary subluxation in children. Pediatr Emerg Care. 1999;15:25–9.
34. Phillips WA, Hensinger RN. The management of rotatory atlanto-axial subluxation in children. J Bone Joint Surg Am. 1989;71:664–5.
35. Lee C, Woodring JH. Unstable Jefferson variant atlas fractures: an unrecognized cervical injury. AJR Am J Roentgenol. 1992;158:113–8.
36. Smoker WRK, Dolan KD. The "fat" C2: a sign of fracture. AJR Am J Roentgenol. 1987;148:609–14.
37. Bulas DI, Fitz CR, Johnson DL. Traumatic atlanto-occipital dislocation in children. Radiology. 1993; 188:155–8.

38. Cohen A, Hirsch M, Kjatz M, Sofer S. Traumatic atlanto-occipital dislocation in children: review and report of five cases. Pediatr Emerg Care. 1991; 7:24–7.

39. Grabb BC, Frye TA, Hedlund GL, Vaid YN, Grabb PA, Royal SA. MRI diagnosis of suspected atlanto-occipital dissociation in childhood. Pediatr Radiol. 1999;29: 275–81.

40. Harris JH, Carson GC, Wagner LK. Radiologic diagnosis of traumatic occipitovertebral relationships on lateral radiographs of supine subjects. AJR Am J Roentgenol. 1994;162:881–6.

Miscellaneous Cervical Spine Problems

6

Inflammation–Infection

The most common inflammatory processes leading to cervical spine instability are the collagen vascular diseases [1, 2], primarily rheumatoid arthritis. These conditions lead to ligament instability, which most often, as far as the cervical spine is concerned, involves the upper and lower portions of the spine. Initially, the apophyseal joints are involved, with the joint space first becoming indistinct and then obliterated (Fig. 6.1a). Later, as the disease process progresses, fusion of the apophyseal joints and indeed, the posterior elements of the cervical vertebra, can occur (Fig. 6.1b). This is most likely to occur with Still's disease, the most aggressive form of rheumatoid arthritis. In the upper cervical spine, atlantoaxial instability also can be seen, and it results in marked displacement of C1 on C2 (Fig. 6.1c).

Osteomyelitis–diskitis of the cervical spine is not as common as it is in the thoracic and lumbar portions of the spine in children. In the lumbar spine, the infection usually is secondary to *Staphylococcus aureus* infection. This problem, however, basically does not occur in the cervical spine. In the thoracic spine, tuberculous infections are more common; but once again, the problem is uncommon in children. Nonetheless, when these infections occur there is destruction of the involved intervertebral disk space, along with bony resorption and destruction of the adjacent vertebral end plates. As a result, the disk space narrows, the end plates become indistinct, and loss of bony substance occurs. In other more common cases there is extensive destruction of the vertebra and in some cases associated destruction of the apophyseal joints (Fig. 6.2). With bacterial and tuberculous infections, disk space narrowing secondary to disk and bony destruction is common, but with fungal disease the disk often is preserved. Osteomylitis can involve the vertebral body, the dens [3], or the neural arch [4].

Another inflammatory condition of the cervical spine is the so-called "calcific diskitis of childhood" [3, 5–7]. This condition, of unknown etiology, but perhaps of viral origin [8], results in inflammation of the intervertebral disks and subsequent calcification. It is attended with pain but is self-limiting. In the early stages the disk spaces are enlarged and bulged [9]. This is best demonstrated with magnetic resonance imaging (Fig. 6.3a, b), but eventually these disks undergo degeneration and calcification. Such calcification, of course, is readily visible on plain films (Fig. 6.3c). It can occur at multiple levels, and also can be seen in the thoracic spine. These disks also can herniate both anteriorly and posteriorly [10], but seldom is neurologic deficit attendant. Because the condition is self-limiting, it requires only supportive, anti-inflammatory, and analgesic therapy.

L.E. Swischuk, *Imaging of the Cervical Spine in Children*,
DOI 10.1007/978-1-4614-3788-8_6, © Springer Science+Business Media New York 2013

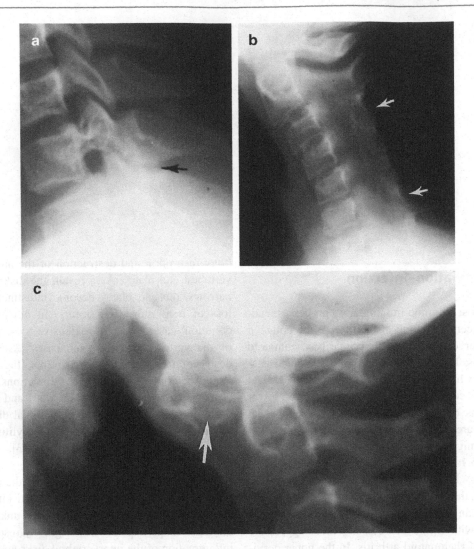

Fig. 6.1 Rheumatoid arthritis. (**a**) Note obliteration of the apophyseal joint (*arrow*) in the lower cervical spine. (**b**) In this patient with Still's disease there is complete fusion of the posterior elements of the cervical spine (*arrows*).

The apophyseal joints are completely obliterated. (**c**) C1–C2 dislocation with marked increase in the predental distance (*arrow*)

Neoplastic Diseases; Malignant and Benign

For the most part, benign tumors or tumorlike lesions consist of hemangiomas, aneurysmal bone cysts, and the occasional osteoid osteoma [11–14]. Hemangiomas characteristically produce a multiloculated expansile lesion, more often involving the posterior elements. However, vertebral body involvement also can occur (Fig. 6.4). Aneurysmal

bone cysts appear much as they do in other portions of the skeleton and spine, producing lytic, slightly expansile, unless compression fractures supervene, lesions of the vertebral body (Fig. 6.5).

Hemangiomas can be differentiated from aneurysmal bone cysts more clearly with MR than with CT imaging. With tomography the multiloculated nature and the primary location of the lesion, of course, are readily demonstrable, but it is with magnetic resonance imaging that differentiation between the two is more definitive.

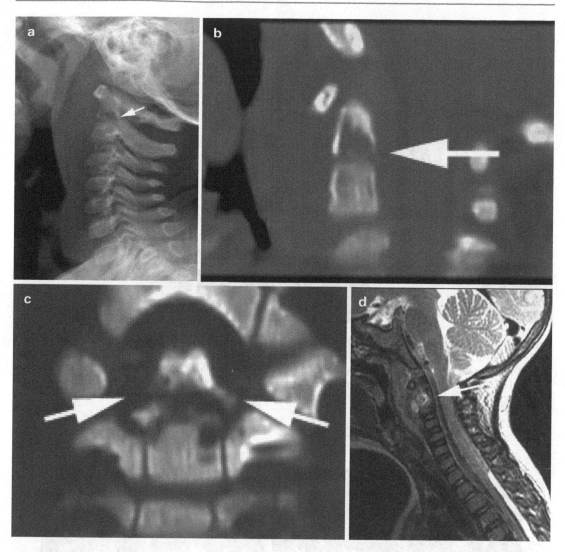

Fig. 6.2 Infection; osteomyelitis. (**a**) Osteomyelitis of C2. Note destruction of the body and dens of C2 (*arrow*). There is pronounced prevertebral soft tissue swelling. (**b**) Sagittal reconstructed CT demonstrates the destruction (*arrow*). (**c**) Coronal reconstructed CT demonstrates destruction of the dens and the body of C2 (*arrows*). (**d**) Sagittal MR, T2-weighted study demonstrates increased signal in the area of osteomyelitis (*arrow*)

The reason for this is that hemangiomas retain high signal on T2-weighted sequences, while aneurysmal bone cysts produce heterogeneous signal. More importantly, however, aneurysmal bone cysts demonstrate pathognomonic blood–fluid levels (Fig. 6.5d). This generally is not seen with any other tumor or cystic bone disease.

Osteoid osteomas, of course, appear as they do at other sites in the spine. They produce sclerosis of the body or pedicle. Rarely, giant osteoid osteomas can be encountered (osteoblastomas).

Similarly, one can occasionally encounter other benign tumors, such as chondromas, various fibrous tumors, and fibrous dysplasia.

Primary malignant tumors of the cervical spine also are very rare, except perhaps for Ewing's sarcoma. The findings of these tumors are similar to those seen elsewhere in the skeleton and the vertebral column. Basically, in the spine they consist of the presence of a destructive lesion in the vertebral body with preservation of the adjacent intervertebral disk space. Most often,

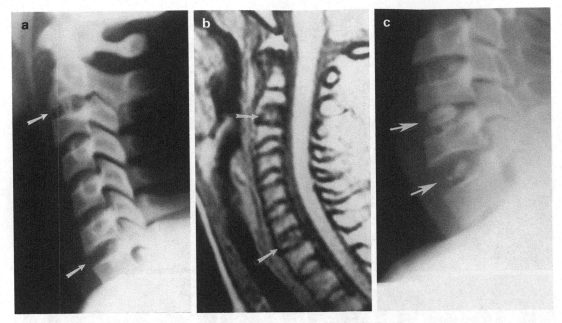

Fig. 6.3 Calcific diskitis. (**a**) Note a slight bulging configuration of two intervertebral disks (*arrows*). (**b**) Loss of signal in the two involved disks (*arrows*) is demonstrated by MRI. This patient also had calcification of an upper thoracic disk. (**c**) Typical calcified disks (*arrows*).

Note the biconcave bulging configuration of the disk spaces ((**a**, **b**) Reproduced with permission from Swischuk LE, Stansberry SD. Calcific discitis: MRI changes in disks without visible calcification. Pediatric Radiology. 1991;21:365–6)

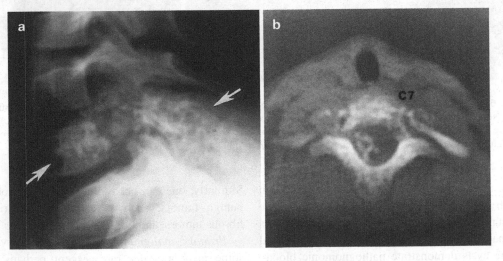

Fig. 6.4 Hemangioma. (**a**) Note the multiloculated, expansile, mixed lytic, and blastic appearance of this hemangioma, which extends from the vertebral body into

the neural arch (*arrows*). (**b**) Axial CT study demonstrates the same findings

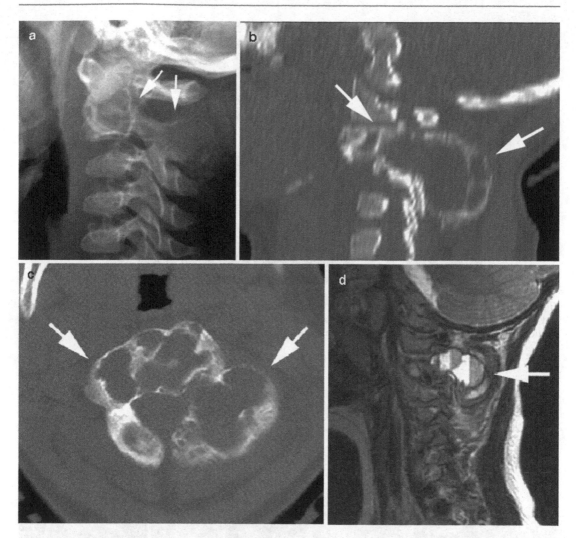

Fig. 6.5 Aneurysmal bone cyst. (**a**) Note the expansile lytic lesion involving the body and neural arch of C2 (*arrows*). (**b**) Sagittal reconstructed CT study demonstrates the same findings (*arrows*). (**c**) Axial CT demonstrates the expanding multiloculated nature of the lesion (*arrows*). (**d**) MR sagittal T2-weighted image demonstrates classic blood–fluid levels within the lesion (*arrow*)

Ewing's sarcoma involves the body of the vertebra, but the posterior elements of the vertebra also can be involved. Ewing's sarcoma can also be multicentric, and in these cases it is difficult to determine whether the lesion truly is multicentric or is metastatic. In either case, however, one can encounter lytic or sclerotic lesions (Fig. 6.6).

Bony involvement of the cervical spine with lymphoma and leukemia is rather uncommon.

Metastatic disease, however, is more common and most often is due to metastatic neuroblastoma. In such cases there is destruction of the vertebral body with loss of vertebral height. The neural arches also can be involved, and pathologic fractures are common. Of course, the findings are not specific for neuroblastoma, for they can be seen with any number of malignant tumors (Fig. 6.7).

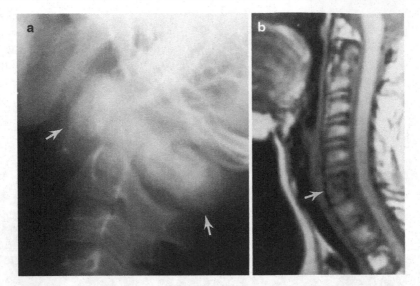

Fig. 6.6 Ewing's sarcoma. (**a**) C1 is markedly expanded and sclerotic (*arrows*) in this patient with metastatic or multicentric Ewing's sarcoma. (**b**) Another patient. Magnetic resonance T1-weighted image demonstrates loss of signal in a vertebral body (*arrow*) involved with metastatic Ewing's tumor

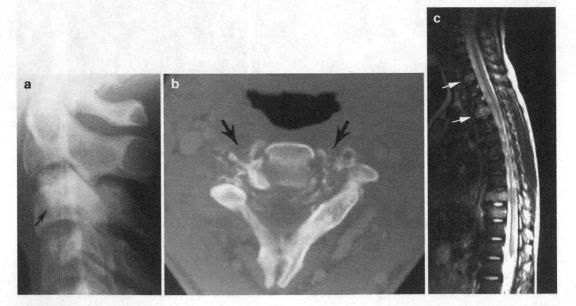

Fig. 6.7 Metastatic disease. (**a**) Note vague sclerosis of the body of C3 (*arrow*) in this patient with metastatic osteogenic sarcoma. (**b**) CT demonstrates the destructive nature of the metastatic lesion (*arrows*). (**c**) Another patient with metastatic rhabdomyosarcoma. On this sagittal T2-weighted MR image note increased signal in a cervical vertebral body (*upper arrow*) and an upper thoracic vertebral body (*lower arrow*). Two other vertebra are involved in the lower thoracic spine with associated pathologic compression

Spinal Cord Tumors and Other Expanding Lesions

Spinal cord tumors generally are rare, and when encountered usually are astrocytomas [15]. Syringomyelia is more common and can be seen as an isolated lesion or perhaps more commonly in association with Arnold-Chiari I malformations [16, 17]. Arachnoid cysts also can occur in the cervical spine but generally are uncommon. Any of these lesions, if present long enough, can produce widening of the spinal canal (Fig. 6.8). However, in the current age, patients come to the attention of physicians much earlier and these bony vertebral changes are seldom seen, and all of these lesions are now best demonstrated with CT or MR imaging (Fig. 6.8) [18].

Neurofibromatosis

The vertebral column notoriously is involved with neurofibromatosis type I [19–22]. The primary problem is bone dysplasia, and in the spine this can be manifest in dysplastic posterior neural arches and vertebral bodies, increased anterior and posterior vertebral body scalloping [19], and enlargement of the intervertebral foramina (due to neurofibromas, or more often dilatation of the subarachnoid space around the nerve roots). Plain films often are the first to reveal these abnormalities, but eventually the entire complex is studied with CT and MR imaging (Fig. 6.9). When plexiform neurofibromatosis is present, extensive, often multilobulated, soft tissue tumors are seen. Frequently these lesions extend into the spinal canal and involve the spinal cord (Fig. 6.10a, b). When the

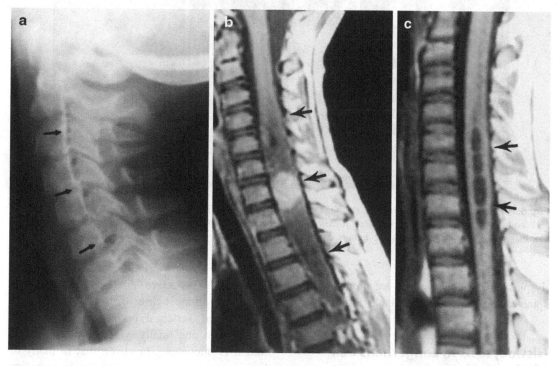

Fig. 6.8 Intraspinal expanding lesions. (**a**) Note the widened spinal canal in this patient with a long-standing glioma. (**b**) MR study in another patient demonstrates increased signal in an extensive glioma (*arrows*), which is causing slight expansion of the cervical canal and obliteration of the cervical spine fluid around the cord. Centrally the high-signal area probably represents concentrated proteinaceous material within a cyst. (**c**) Multiple central cysts (*arrows*) in a patient with syringomyelia. Note that the spinal cord is slightly widened in the area of involvement

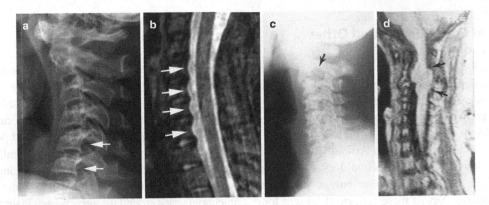

Fig. 6.9 Neurofibromatosis. (**a**) Note increased vertebral scalloping in two lower cervical vertebral bodies (*arrows*). This was an incidental finding. (**b**) Sagittal MR T2-weighted study demonstrates increased posterior scalloping with increase in the subarachnoid space at multiple levels (*arrows*). (**c**) Another patient. Note the markedly dysplastic vertebral bodies demonstrating both anterior and posterior concave scalloping. The intervertebral foramen between C2 and C3 is markedly enlarged (*arrow*). (**d**) Same patient demonstrating a glioma (*arrows*) of the spinal cord in the area of the enlarged neural foramen

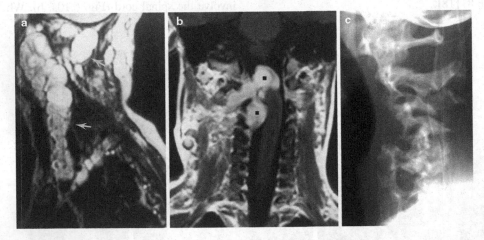

Fig. 6.10 Plexiform neurofibromatosis. (**a**) Note extensive nodular tumors throughout the neck (*arrows*). (**b**) Coronal MR study demonstrates the tumors extending into the spinal canal (*squares*). (**c**) Another patient whose plain films show a grossly distorted and dysplastic cervical spine

dysplastic vertebral changes are pronounced the spine can become grossly unstable (Fig. 6.10c).

Histiocytosis X; Langerhans Cell Histiocytosis

Histiocytosis X, or Langerhans cell histiocytosis, is a very common condition in childhood [23]. It frequently involves the spine, and cervical spine involvement is common. Classically the abnormality involves the vertebral body, although the spinous processes also can be involved (Fig. 6.11). In most cases there is destruction of the involved vertebral body with progressive compression and finally, vertebra plana formation. It is interesting, however, that in many of these cases, even though compression is extensive, there is very little in the way of paraspinal hematoma or soft tissue mass formation (Fig. 6.11). When the findings are advanced, pathologic dislocation can be seen (Fig. 6.11) but the intervertebral disk spaces usually are preserved, and in this regard, the findings must be

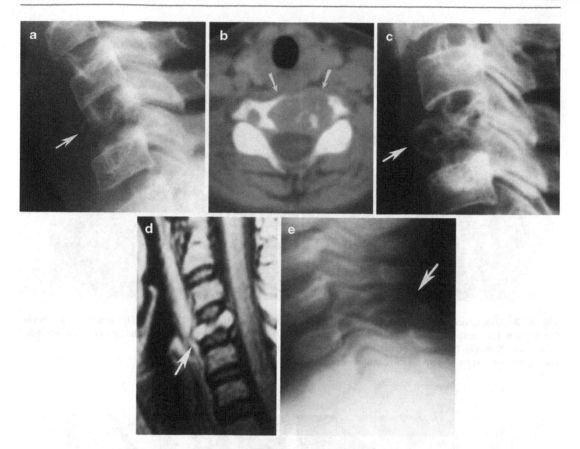

Fig. 6.11 Histiocytosis X. (**a**) Note destruction of the vertebral body (*arrow*). There is slight dislocation present. (**b**) CT study demonstrates nonspecific lytic destruction of the vertebral body (*arrows*). Note however, that there is very little, if any, soft tissue component. (**c**) Another patient with similar destruction of a vertebral body (*arrow*). (**d**) MR study, T1 weighted, demonstrates the collapsed vertebral body, which is protruding both anteriorly and posteriorly (*arrow*). Signal within the body is normal. (**e**) In this patient destruction involves the neural arch only (*arrow*)

differentiated from those of metastatic or other tumoral destruction of the vertebral bodies. It is helpful, of course, if other characteristic skeletal lesions are present in these patients. CT and MR images also are excellent in demonstrating the abnormal findings but provide little in the way of differentiating information (Fig. 6.11).

also be seen in normal individuals, as an isolated phenomenon. Interestingly enough, however, even though the findings may be dramatic, especially on flexion–extension views of the cervical spine (Fig. 6.12), neurologic deficit is seldom present [24, 25]. In a few cases, however, this may not be true [29].

Atlanto-Occipital Instability

Traumatic atlanto-occipital disruption usually is seen with severe cervical spine injuries, and the patient often is dead on arrival to the emergency room. Chronic atlanto-occipital instability is another problem and most commonly is seen on a congenital basis in trisomy 21 [24–28]. It can

Spinal Stenosis

Spinal stenosis can occur anywhere throughout the vertebral column. Most often it occurs at lower levels, but it is sometimes observed in the cervical spine. The spinal canal is narrower than normal, and the scant subarachnoid space is readily demonstrable with MR imaging (Fig. 6.13).

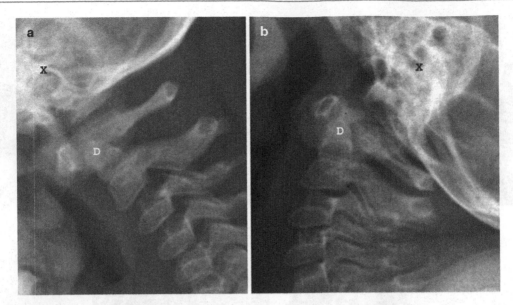

Fig. 6.12 Atlanto-occipital instability. (**a**) Trisomy 21. On flexion the dens (D) lines up normally with the calvarium. X marks the center of the mastoid/petruous bone complex. (**b**) On extension the occiput is markedly posteriorly displaced. The dens (D) now lies far anterior to the occiput. X again marks the center of the mastoid/petrous bone complex

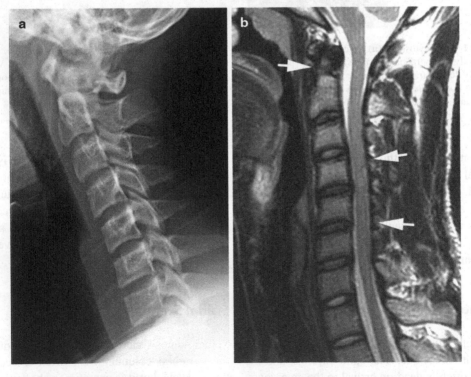

Fig. 6.13 Spinal stenosis. (**a**) Plain films of the cervical spine are normal except that the spinal canal appears a little narrow. (**b**) MR sagittal T2-weighted study demonstrates the tight canal (*arrows*) obliterating the subarachnoid space and with the bony canal in close apposition to the spinal cord

References

1. Babini SM, Cocco JA, Babini JC, et al. Atlantoaxial subluxation in systemic lupus erythematosus: further evidence of tendinous alterations. J Rheumatol. 1990;17:173–7.
2. Reid GD, Hill RH. Atlantoaxial subluxation in juvenile ankylosing spondylitis. J Pediatr. 1978;93:531–2.
3. Nolting L, Singer J, Hackett R, Kleiner L. Acute hematogenous osteomyelitis of the odontoid process in a child with torticollis. Pediatr Emerg Care. 2010;26:669–71.
4. Reiss-Zimmermann M, Hirsch W, Schuster V, Wojan M, Sorge I. Pyogenic osteomyelitis of the vertebral arch in children. J Pediatr Surg. 2010;45:1737–40.
5. Girodias J-B, Azouz EM, Maarton D. Intervertebral disk space calcification. A report of 51 children with a review of the literature. Pediatr Radiol. 1991;21: 541–6.
6. Heinrich SD, Zembo MM, King AG, et al. Calcific cervical intervertebral disk herniation in children. Spine. 1991;16:228–31.
7. McGregor JC, Butler P. Disk calcification in childhood computed tomographic and magnetic resonance imaging appearances. Br J Radiol. 1986;59:180.
8. Swischuk LE, Junag M, Jadhav SP. Calcific discitis in children: vertebral body involvement (possible insight into etiology). Emerg Radiol. 2008;15(6):427–30.
9. Swischuk LE, Stansberry SD. Calcific discitis: MRI changes in disks without visible calcification. Pediatr Radiol. 1991;21:365–6.
10. Sutton TJ, Turcotte B. Posterior herniation of calcified intervertebral discs in children. J Can Assoc Radiol. 1973;24:131–6.
11. Azouz EM, Kozlowski K, Marton D, et al. Osteoid osteoma and osteoblastoma of the spine in children. Pediatr Radiol. 1986;16:25–31.
12. Caro PA, Mandell GA, Stanton RP. Aneurysmal bone cyst of the spine in children. MRI imaging at 0.5 tesla. Pediatr Radiol. 1991;21:117–20.
13. Kozlowski K, Beluffi G, Masel J, et al. Primary vertebral tumours in children. Report of 20 cases with brief literature review. Pediatr Radiol. 1984;14:129–39.
14. Myles ST, MacRae ME. Benign osteoblastoma of the spine in childhood. J Neurosurg. 1988;68:884–8.
15. Umemoto M, Azuma E, Ohshima S, et al. Congenital astrocytoma in the cervical spinal cord. Am J Dis Child. 1990;144:744–6.
16. Dure LS, Percy AK, Cheek WR, et al. Chiari type I malformation in children. J Pediatr. 1989;114:573–6.
17. Elster AD, Chen MYM. Chiari I malformations: clinical and radiological reappraisal. Radiology. 1992;183: 347–53.
18. Lee BCP, Zimmerman RD, Manning JJ. MR imaging of syringomyelia and hydromyelia. Am J Neuroradiol. 1985;6:221–6.
19. Casselman ES, Mandell GA. Vertebral scalloping in neurofibromatosis. Radiology. 1979;131:89–94.
20. Leeds NE, Jacobson HG. Spinal neurofibromatosis. Am J Roentgenol. 1976;126:617–23.
21. Sirois III JL, Drennan JC. Dystrophic spinal deformity in neurofibromatosis. J Pediatr Orthop. 1990;10: 522–6.
22. Yaghmai I. Spine changes in neurofibromatosis. Radiographics. 1986;6:261–85.
23. Meyer JS, Harty MP, Mahboubi S, et al. Langerhans' cell histiocytosis: presentation and evolution of radiologic findings with clinical correlation. Radiographics. 1995;15:1135–46.
24. Davidson RG. Atlantoaxial instability in individuals with Down syndrome: a fresh look at the evidence. Pediatrics. 1988;81:857–65.
25. Babini SM, Maldonado Cocco JA, El-Khoury CY, et al. Posterior atlanto-occipital subluxation in Down syndrome. Radiology. 1986;159:507–9.
26. Herring JA, Fielding JW. Cervical instability in Down's syndrome and juvenile rheumatoid arthritis. J Pediatr Orthop. 1982;2:205–7.
27. Hungerford GD, Akkaraju V, Rawe SE, et al. Atlanto-occipital and atlantoaxial dislocations with spinal cord compression in Downs syndrome: a case report and review of the literature. Br J Radiol. 1981;54: 758–61.
28. Stein SM, Kirchner SG, Horev G, et al. Atlanto-occipital subluxation in Down syndrome. Pediatr Radiol. 1991;21:121–4.
29. Bhatnagar M, Sponseller PD, Carroll IV C, et al. Pediatric atlantoaxial instability presenting as cerebral and cerebellar infarcts. J Pediatr Orthop. 1991;11: 103–7.

Index

L.E. Swischuk, *Imaging of the Cervical Spine in Children*,
DOI 10.1007/978-1-4614-3788-8, © Springer Science+Business Media New York 2013

Printed in the United States
By Bookmasters